Eliciting Care

New Perspectives in Southeast Asian Studies

Eliciting Care

Health and Power in Northern Thailand

Bo Kyeong Seo

THE UNIVERSITY OF WISCONSIN PRESS

The University of Wisconsin Press
728 State Street, Suite 443
Madison, Wisconsin 53706
uwpress.wisc.edu

Gray's Inn House, 127 Clerkenwell Road
London ECIR 5DB, United Kingdom
eurospanbookstore.com

Printed in the United States of America
This book may be available in a digital edition.

Library of Congress Cataloging-in-Publication Data

Names: Seo, Bo Kyeong, author.
Title: Eliciting care : health and power in northern Thailand / Bo Kyeong Seo.
Other titles: New perspectives in Southeast Asian studies.
Description: Madison, Wisconsin : The University of Wisconsin Press, [2020] |
Series: New perspectives in Southeast Asian studies |
Includes bibliographical references and index.
Identifiers: LCCN 2019041272 | ISBN 9780299326906 (hardback)
Subjects: LCSH: Medical care—Thailand, Northern. | Medical anthropology—Thailand, Northern. | Health services accessibility—Thailand, Northern. | Caregivers—Thailand, Northern.
Classification: LCC GN296.5.T5 S46 2020 | DDC 362.109593—dc23
LC record available at https://lccn.loc.gov/2019041272

For my parents

~

For Philip

CONTENTS

List of Illustrations ix
Acknowledgments xi

Introduction: Others' Unpleasant Feet 3
1 The Government of Care 23
2 Patient Waiting 39
3 Careful Inscription 58
4 Premature Life and Death 78
5 Vulnerability and Nurturance at Home 94
6 Spirits and the Circuitry of Care 118
Conclusion: An Affirmative Politics of Care 140

Notes 149
References 163
Index 181

ILLUSTRATIONS

Maps

Map of Thailand in the region xvi
Map of Shan State in the region xvii

Photos

Different forms of identification for non-Thai citizens 62
A self-diagnosis table for postpartum depression 71
Birth documents 72
Antenatal care logbook 75
The altar for Aunt Uan 123
A picture of a Shan prince 126
Praying at a shrine for spirits 131
Healing chants 133

Tables

Table 1. Total visits to Ban Phaet Hospital antenatal care from October 2007 to September 2010 64
Table 2. Number of antenatal care visits in Ban Phaet Hospital from October 2007 to September 2010 65
Table 3. Timing of first antenatal visit, Ban Phaet Hospital Antenatal Clinic, October 2007 to September 2010 66

ACKNOWLEDGMENTS

This book is about how people care for each other. I myself was the recipient of thoughtful care and nurturing while researching and writing this study, and I would like to extend my heartfelt thanks, first and foremost, to the doctors, nurses, nurses' aides, administrative staff, and patients at Ban Phaet Hospital who accommodated me over several years. Though I am not able to list their real names here, their struggles, passions, and hopes resonate throughout this book. Their invaluable help and support made it possible for me to think about and experience care in unaccustomed ways. I also want to express my deepest gratitude to the Shan women for sharing their stories, even in very difficult moments of their lives. One of my Shan sisters, Sen, once told me that she hoped that my anthropological work would allow people she would never meet to know about her life. It was an honor and great fortune to be trusted with these stories, and I hope that this book fulfills her wish.

I also want to express my profound gratitude to the many people whom I came to know, rely on, and learn from in Chiang Mai. The Duwangrat family allowed me to stay in their home during my fieldwork and provided the great warmth of a big extended family, which I had never experienced before. My aunt Thi, who never married but raised many children, including me, always knew when I was feeling low and lifted me up with her fluffy omelets and tender cheer. The Regional Center for Social Science and Sustainable Development at Chiang Mai University also offered me an academic home for many years, and this book owes much to their support.

I thank Chayan Vaddhanaphuti, Malee Sittikreangkrai, Amporn Jirattikorn, Aranya Siriphon, and several RCSD administrative staff members for their support and hospitality. I also owe special thanks to Arunrat Tangmunkongvorakul and Linda Aurpibul at the Research Institute for Health Science for teaching me a great deal about the Thai public health system and neonatal medicine. Several talented young researchers from Chiang Mai University helped me with transcribing recordings and navigating villages and construction sites: Busarin Lertchavalitsakul, Mim Kasama, May Wannalak, and especially Thirayut Sangangamsakun and Sai Loung were indispensable parts of my life in Chiang Mai as creative research collaborators, patient language teachers, and great drinking buddies all at once. Without their treasured friendship, fieldwork would have been much less enjoyable.

This book could not have been written without the continuing support of all my mentors, colleagues, and friends. I am deeply grateful to Philip Taylor for his brilliant insights and boundless encouragement. My thinking benefited very much from his invaluable gifts of input, challenging questions, and confidence in this project. He has read more versions of this manuscript than anyone would wish to and has been a trusted source of advice. During my doctoral years at the Australian National University, I also received essential guidance and support from Kathryn Robinson, Andrew Walker, Andrew Kipnis, the late Nicholas Tapp, Peter Jackson, and Tyrell Haberkorn. My peers at Canberra—Geoff Buchanan, Gillian Dalgetty, Preedee Hongsaton, Visisya Pinthongvijayakul, Tanisha Jowsey, Zhuzhu, and Emilie Ens—also provided much valued friendship and inspiration.

I am also very fortunate to have been a part of several vigorous communities of scholars who enriched this book with conversations, debates, and friendship. I was lucky to join the Medical Anthropology Summer School organized by the Institute of Social and Cultural Anthropology, Freie Universität Berlin, in 2013. This experience greatly expanded my understanding of medical anthropology and global health. I am especially grateful to Pierre Minn, Nolan Kline, and Heide Castañeda for their encouragement and advice. My acquaintances with anthropologists based in Berlin deepened into friendships when I joined the institute as a postdoctoral fellow. I would like to thank Hansjörg Dilger for his thoughtful mentoring and support and the members of the medical anthropology group for their warm hospitality and intellectual stimulation. Roberta Zavoretti, Anika Koenig, and Britta Rutert made my years in Berlin much happier. At Thammasat University, I owe a debt of gratitude to the Faculty of Sociology and Anthropology, especially to Prasert Langkla and Boonlert Visetpricha. In Seoul, Myung Seok Oh, Su Hong Chae, and Yun Hwan Shin, who sparked my interest in Southeast Asian studies, have offered much encouragement during the various stages of this book project. My colleagues at Yonsei University, especially Hyun Mi Kim, Sang Kok Lee, and Mun Young Cho, have been incredibly supportive during the completion of the manuscript.

It has been a pleasure and honor to work with the University of Wisconsin Press. I thank Gwen Walker for her guidance and steadfast support for this project, Sheila McMahon for effectively guiding the manuscript to completion, and Judith Robey for careful copyediting. I am also deeply grateful to two anonymous reviewers and to series editor Katherine Bowie, whose encouraging and thorough feedback helped the manuscript immensely and breathed new life into the project. Theodore Jun Yoo and Michale Herzfeld provided helpful advice on publishing, and Ji Eun Kim offered a close reading of the introduction in the manuscript's later stages.

The research on which this book is based would not have been possible without the generous institutional support that I have received over the years. Grants from the Australian National University and the Asia Institute at the University of Melbourne (a Thai Studies Field Research Grant) enabled me to conduct my initial fieldwork and to write up the results. I also was awarded an ENITS Scholarship from the Institute of Thai Studies at Chulalongkorn University and the Sir Raymond Firth Award from the Department of Anthropology at ANU. I am particularly grateful for the German Research Foundation for a Dahlem Research School POINT Fellowship, which allowed me to organized follow-up visits and to spend time on revisions. The final writing phase for this book was supported in part by the Yonsei University Future-Leading Research Initiative (2018-22-0101).

Earlier versions of parts of chapter 2 appeared in the article "Patient Waiting: Care as a Gift and Debt in the Thai Healthcare System," *Journal of Royal Anthropological Institute* 22 (2): 279–95. A version of chapter 3 appeared in the article "Caring for Premature Life and Death: The Relational Dynamics of Detachment in a NICU," *Medical Anthropology* 35 (6): 560–71, while a version of chapter 4 appeared in the article "The Work of

Inscription: Antenatal Care, Birth Documents, and Shan Migrant Women in Chiang Mai," *Medical Anthropology Quarterly* 31 (4): 481–98.

My parents, Young Ok Eo and Jong Seok Seo, who have anxiously awaited the completion of this book, continue to inspire me to be adventurous both in life and writing. Finally, Su Kyeong Kim's love and care has enriched all parts of this book.

NOTE ON TRANSLITERATION

Unless stated otherwise, all translations in this book are mine. I follow a modified version of the Royal Thai General System of Transcription. The RTGST makes no distinction between long and short vowel forms, and tones are not represented. The modified system I adopt in this book differs from the RTGST in two ways. First, although the RTGST does not differentiate the aspirated and unaspirated forms of *ch*, I render the unaspirated form as *j*. Second, while in the RTGST *o* is used for the central, unrounded vowel in Thai, I replace it with *oh*. For example, *oh* in *moh* (doctor) represents the sound of the "aw" in "law" as it is pronounced in American standard usage or the "ore" in "more" as it is pronounced in British/Australian standard usage. My intention is to increase the plausibility of a non-Thai speaker's attempt to pronounce the Thai expressions given in this book. I have not changed the words and names that have acquired a familiar romanized form, such as the Thai currency (baht), as well as proper names that individuals have transliterated themselves. I also follow the Thai norm of referring to Thai authors by first names, and all citations by Thai authors are in alphabetical order in the bibliography according to first names.

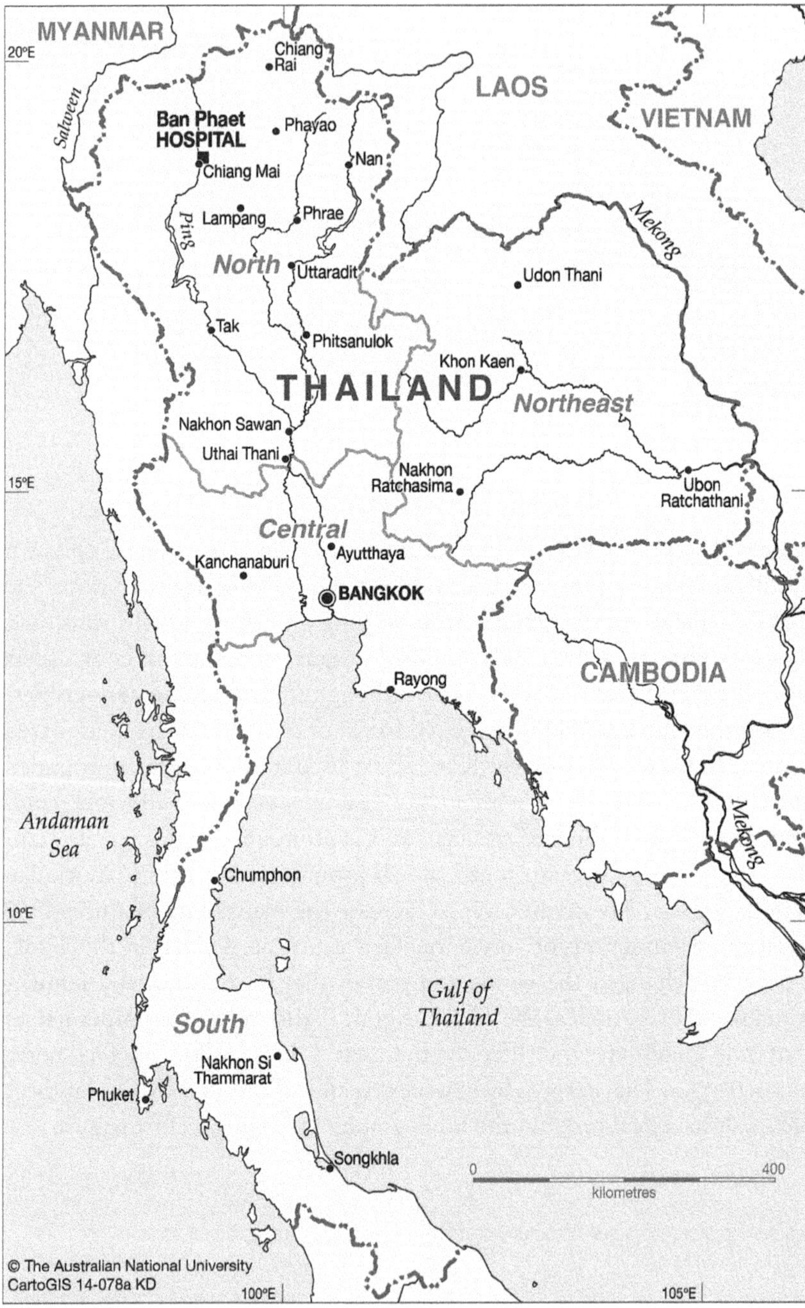

Figure 1. Map of Thailand in the region

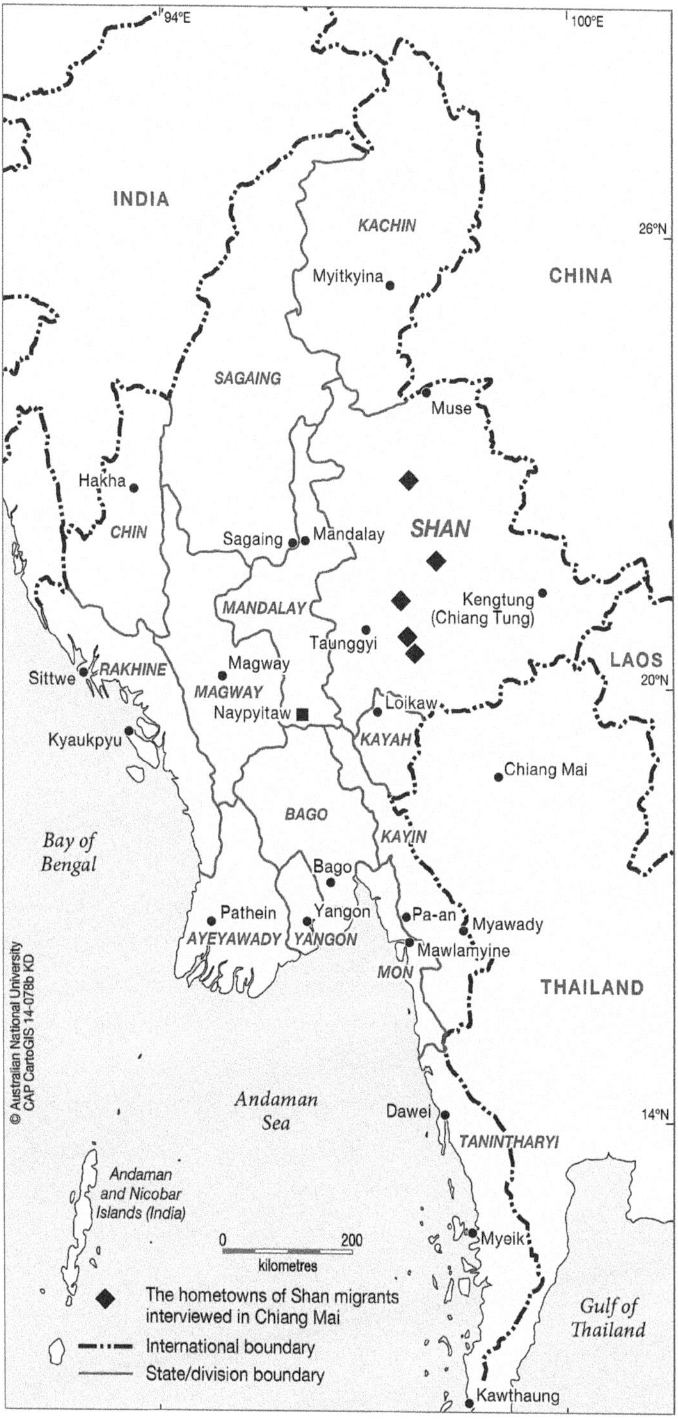

Figure 2. Map of Shan State in the region

Eliciting Care

Introduction

Others' Unpleasant Feet

As I sat on a plastic chair between Uncle Bun's and Ek's beds in Ban Phaet Hospital, located in a semirural community in Chiang Mai, in northern Thailand, I could not help noticing the patients' feet poking out from under the bed sheets. Uncle Bun, a seventy-five-year-old Thai man, had been immobile for three years, and the flesh on his bony and pale feet was dying. Prolonged bed rest had caused severe pressure sores, and his feet had lost their ability to move and were becoming gangrenous. On the other side of me, Ek's feet were dusky, toughened, and unwashed. A young Shan laborer, Ek had been paralyzed and was barely conscious after a motorbike accident. The tall and strong man's huge feet were stained by blackish oil and blood. Although he had been in the intensive care unit (ICU) for two weeks before he was transferred to this ward, no one had washed the bloodstains from his feet. His broken toenails were covered in dirt, and the skin on his heels was cracked. I first met these bed-ridden patients in August 2010, and for a month-long period of hospitalization these men's feet never touched the ground.

I often sat between the two men at their relatives' invitation. Aunt Deng, Uncle Bun's wife, told me several things about him while spending all day at his bedside. Uncle Bun was born in Chiang Mai and had lived his whole life in a village near the hospital, working as a day laborer. The couple's two sons had died young. Uncle Bun had developed paralysis three years ago, and Aunt Deng had taken care of him by herself. The only income for this tiny family was a pension for two, at 1,000 baht (around USD 30) per month. Sitting beside Ek was his sister Phon, who was in her late twenties. After all the siblings in their family had moved to Chiang Mai from Shan State in Burma, she had almost lost touch with her older brother. Then, his sudden injury reunited them. Ek was found unconscious on the roadside, and it was a community hospital nurse who traced Ek's information on his work permit and contacted the village leader at his registered address. The village leader made some inquiries, and weeks later Ek's estranged brothers and sisters gathered around his hospital bed. Phon had not seen her brother for seven years but now stayed with him almost every day.

The effect of Phon's presence showed immediately in Ek's feet: upon her arrival she washed the blood away and trimmed her brother's dirty toenails. She helped the nurses' aides when they changed his diaper and linens, and she soon began providing most of his daily care. The ward nurses complimented Phon, saying she was a *khon di* (virtuous person) who did not abandon her unfortunate brother despite her difficult situation. Yet to me Phon's exhaustion was evident. As a young mother of a five-year-old son and destitute migrant worker, she had taken on a burden of care that was onerous. Her care of Ek meant that the family had to live solely on her husband's meager income. Phon was much relieved that the cost of Ek's treatment would be covered by health insurance for migrant workers, but just making the daily trip to the hospital and back had already strained her family's tight budget. As she once told me while cleaning the phlegm from Ek's breathing tube, "Life is hard. Really hard."

Aunt Deng, meanwhile, was struggling to help care for Uncle Bun's left foot. She had been told to change his position every four hours and give him regular leg massages. But although the ward staff were concerned about the increasing size of the ulcers on his foot, she was reluctant to follow their instructions. She thought that all these unnecessary movements only caused him more pain. The nurse warned her several times that if the sores got worse, he would need further surgery. The subtle tension between Aunt Deng and the ward nurses intensified when she requested an end to his nasal tube feedings because she felt that putting liquid food through his nose with a syringe was hurting her husband. Yet the ward nurses could not honor her request. One nurse explained, "His pneumonia is gone now. He is really weak from not eating. After we started tube feeding, he gained more strength. If we are not doing anything to help the patient, there is no reason for him to be in the hospital. She cannot just wait here until he dies." Finally, the nurse reported the feeding issue to the attending physician and delivered the final message that if Deng wanted to stop tube feeding, then the hospital had to discharge him. For Aunt Deng, that was not something she could cope with: "I can't take care of him at home all alone. We have to be here. I don't know how long I will suffer here, but what can I do?" she told me with a tired smile. Both parties wanted to provide comfort for the dying man, but they seemed to take different positions concerning the kind of care he needed.

One evening a welcome visitor finally arrived in the ward to see Uncle Bun: Ajan Ruam, a traditional doctor (*moh boran*) whom Aunt Deng had repeatedly invited. As she had requested, the *moh boran* organized a brief ritual called *su khwan* at his bedside. A boat-shaped banana leaf containing *jampi* (magnolia) flowers, a small candle, *khaep mu* (fried pork cracklings), and sticky rice—a staple of the northern Thai diet—was set above the patient's head as an offering for the protective spirits. The traditional doctor then tied a thick white cotton string around Uncle Bun's wrist and whispered sacred words. Aunt Deng explained to me that this brief ritual would anchor Uncle Bun's soul into his body and therefore make him well. The quiet rite smoothly blended into the evening rhythm of the ward. A couple of days later, the attending physician again removed the dead and decaying tissue from Uncle Bun's foot.

From time to time, I again caught a glimpse of these men's feet. Uncle Bun's foot, damaged by pressure from the weight of his own body, stiff and bloodless, foretold his imminent death. On the other side, Ek's feet reflected some improvement in his state: absolute bedrest during his month-long period of hospitalization had freed Ek from hard manual labor, and this change could be seen in his feet, which no longer bore witness to his life of toil. The skin had softened, and the cracks on the skin of his heels had started to close. When Ek suddenly dropped his foot from the bed, Phon and I could see dead skin floating in the rays of the afternoon sunlight. We had no idea what the outcome of Ek's brain damage would be at that time, but the abrupt movement of his foot clearly showed that he was alive. At the bedside of neighboring patients, pain and worries were not articulated in words. But the two men's mute feet gave eloquent expression to the nature of their grave ailments and the care they were receiving.

How we as humans respond to others' need for care, especially in times of disruption associated with disease and impairment, is the subject of this book. I have begun with the disfigured feet of Ek and Uncle Bun because they strike me as emblematic of the regimes of care in which both men were ensnared and because the prominent display of these two sets of extremities in the hospital ward served to disrupt the symbolic hierarchy central to the Thai conception of the human body. Pointing one's feet at someone is considered rude in Thailand since feet are regarded as the lowest and dirtiest part of the body. By contrast, the head is the most sacred as it occupies the highest place in the body and contains its spiritual essences (*khwan* and *winyan*). However, when illness took away these two men's ability to stand or speak, their bodies' lowest reaches assumed remarkable charisma and eloquence. There was something deeply compelling about the vulnerability and patience expressed in these damaged feet, whose sheer presence spoke not only of human fragility but also of the unexpected force of that fragility. Their troubling and stubborn thereness viscerally challenged others to engage with them.

The people tending to these impaired feet drew my attention as well: these included doctors, nurses, nurses' aides, physical therapists, and family members. While all of them contributed to sustaining these men's lives, they also exuded a sense of urgency as well as weariness as caring for others took its toll on their own lives. Aunt Deng and Phon, in particular, experienced care for sick family members as not only a physical challenge but also a moral one. The quotidian work that these caregivers shouldered threatened not only their own well-being and security but also those of their families, making care not simply a moral good but rather a sometimes ambivalent act that can entail risk and trade-offs.

This book is about the generative and disruptive potentialities of care and how care in all forms—physical, emotional, personal, institutional, biomedical, and spiritual—is elicited in relation to the demands of others' bodies and lives. By showing what work is done in response to affective calls for involvement in the lives of others—calls that are made by the embodied presence of the sick, the infirm, the impaired, and the dying and that compel life-sustaining relations of mutuality—the study affirms an idea of care as a process and outcome of elicitation. Care is a relation of coactivity, constantly being remade by those who participate in it, as opposed to something merely offered, appropriated, experienced, or endured.

This book's journey starts at the frontline of the Thai public health care system, in a district hospital I call Ban Phaet Hospital. As Thailand's universal health coverage promises that all people can access needed health services without experiencing financial hardship, this new social contract is redemptive but at the same time exacerbates existing inequalities. While the rich can avail themselves of private services, avoiding crowded public facilities, poor citizens like Aunt Deng and Phon must learn how to navigate institutional and bureaucratic red tape. Ban Phaet Hospital presents a comprehensive picture of how universal health coverage works as the central hub of care and protection, especially for poor and vulnerable groups in the region. This setting also exemplifies what people, both health care providers and users, do to make this system more reliable. The hospital operates beyond the field of biomedicine, becoming deeply connected to other circuits of care that make life possible under conditions of adversity, scarcity, and dislocation. The stories of this hospital, then, expand into layered narratives about familial and religious practices that draw upon different forms of life-sustaining power. By weaving institutional and personal struggles together, I hope to illuminate dynamic connections between the political economy of health and people's lived experience of care. All these diverse projects of care will reveal how multiple relationalities, human and nonhuman agencies, and unforeseen technologies are assembled by a process that I conceptualize as elicitation.

Multiplicity of Care

Care can mean different things, particularly in different settings. The English-language concept of care entails both an affective state (caring about) and a practical action (caring for). An interesting starting point for this analysis is the fact that this duality of meaning is not sustained in all languages, and particularly not in the two primary languages—Korean and Thai—that are central to my work as a native Korean anthropologist working in Thailand.[1] I will show in the following pages that various Thai concepts and terms do not recognize the same distinction between feeling and action, instead allowing for wider interpretations of the tasks and relations of care and caring than occurs in English.

What is care, where does care come from, who cares, and why? These are questions that feminist scholars in particular have strenuously addressed. A rich literature on care ethics that emerged from feminist philosophy has critically engaged with care as first and foremost "work that makes our lives possible in their very vulnerability" (Ferrarese 2016, 150).[2] During early childhood, at times of illness or impairment, and in old age we all need others' care and help. This shared but not uniform condition of dependence lies at the foundation of human solidarity and social provision.

Feminist philosopher Joan Tronto offers a most extensive definition of care as "everything that we do to maintain, continue and repair our world, so that we can live in it as well as possible in a complex, life sustaining web" (1993, 103).[3] In this tradition, care is *life's work* and plays an important role in producing and reproducing both biological and social life. As care can encompass "wage work, child care, domestic labor, sustenance and repair of community ties" (W. Brown 2004, 197), the problematic is that in capitalist economies such pivotal work of social reproduction is undervalued and stratified along lines of class, gender, and racial inequalities (Glenn 2010).[4]

As indicated in the opening of this introduction, tending to the body, soul, and relationships constitutes the heart of care, which is not so much a subsidiary part of biomedicine as it is a concept that informs the logic of that field of knowledge (Mol 2008). Here it is also crucial to note that the promise of care is not merely a matter of individual practices but is also fundamentally mediated by the state. The public ward with which I began is indeed part and parcel of a biopolitical infrastructure that incorporates biological life into a field of governance. Biopower, as outlined by Michel Foucault, refers to a political technology that "brought life and its mechanisms into the realm of explicit calculations and made knowledge/power an agent of transformation of human life" (1978, 143). The concept of biopolitics allows us to grasp the crucial juncture at which the *management of life* has become integral to the modern state power. Welfare and public health measures like universal health coverage constitute a historical product of biopolitics that takes the temporal process of a population—its reproduction, disease, and mortality—as its object. As biopolitical states are interested in the productivity, development, and quality of their populations, states' interventions in individual and collective life take the form of not only regulation but also care.

One problem with biopolitical care is that it appears rather uncaring as it is based on the unequal distribution of the value of life.[5] One of the key anthropological insights into biopolitics is that while its logic asserts the sacredness of life as an abstract concept, it brings about sacrificial populations whose sufferings and deaths are unacknowledged and tolerated.[6] By critically reexamining the intentions and outcomes of the biopolitical deployment of care, several ethnographic works shed light on how the state's care and protection of certain individuals and groups coexist with the acceptance of suffering and death for others. The paradox is that in its efforts to help the poor, undocumented migrants, refugees, ethnic minorities, and other "unwanted" groups, the state also applies brutal measures of policing and containment in the name of care, compassion, and rescue.[7] In these regimes of biopower, care seems to be "arbitrary in its consequences" at best, as Akhil Gupta suggests in the modern history of poverty relief programs in India (2012, 24). At times care by the state can be fundamentally life-destroying in a sense that not the full personhood of those in pain but only their mere survival as a living being is concerned, as Lisa Stevenson (2014) shows in the case of Canadian bureaucrats' attempts to protect Inuit populations.

Anthropological explorations of biopower have exposed how human life rendered as a biological and statistical entity is managed, controlled, and sustained by a certain regime of power. Given that this particular exercise of power also can turn out to be a form of care, it pushes us to critically engage with the good in care practices. Care can entail moral and ethical values that are closely attached to "sensibilities of empathy, compassion, respect, and love" (Kleinman 2015, 240), yet various practices of care generate rather ambivalent experiences and consequences that do not align with these ideals.[8]

The approach taken in this book is grounded in an attentiveness to this ambivalent dynamic of care. Instead of assuming that the ethics of care is antithetical or irrelevant to the macrosocial scale of biopolitics, this book is concerned with how care finds its ethical and political expressions in conditions of uncertainty and ambiguity. If biopolitical structures for the support of life reorganize the responsibility to care in today's political economy, what happened in a country like Thailand, where political instability has remained a lingering menace? What kinds of care practices are enabled and constrained in a field of biopolitics that retains various uncaring measures? If care is a fluid and conflicting set of relations, how is it brought into effect, and by whom? When life is understood and lived as more than a biological entity but appears to have various forms in the local world, how do the plural conceptions of life alter the meanings and methods of care? By going deeper into the uneven terrains of care, this book offers a new way to understand the interplay of power, sociality, and obligation.

Contentious Politics of Universal Health

This study of care in Thailand is located at a particularly important historical juncture. The global health revolution in Thailand witnessed a country with a gross national income (GNI) of 1,900 US dollars per capita in 2002 providing publicly financed health insurance plans for almost the entire population (Sakolsatayadorn Piyasakol 2016). Thailand's health insurance coverage markedly increased from 70 percent in 2001 to 98 percent of its population by 2009, and 18 million people who had before shouldered out-of-pocket payments began to have health insurance (Viroj Tangcharoensathien et al. 2011, 2014). Considering the fact that 28.5 million people in the United States, 8.8 percent of the total population, were still uninsured in 2017 (Berchick, Hood, and Barnett 2018), Thailand's continuous provision of universal coverage is undoubtedly remarkable. Given this dramatic success, Thailand has taken a leading position in the global debate on the institutionalization of the right to health. For instance, World Bank President Jim Yong Kim praised Thailand's bold decision to launch universal coverage against pessimistic concerns over fiscal sustainability at the World Health Assembly (Kim 2013). Amartya Sen, the Nobel Prize–winning economist, also notes the Thai experience of health insurance reform as an exemplary case that demonstrates that providing affordable health care for every citizen is a fully attainable and requisite goal of many countries in the Global South for the sake of equitable development (Drèze and Sen 2013; Sen 2015).

Although Thailand deserves to be lauded for this achievement, the politics of universal health care is far more complex than is depicted in discussions of sustainable development. Thailand is one of the most inequitable countries in Southeast Asia, renowned for its political instability (Pasuk Phongpaichit and Baker 2016). The first ten years of universal health coverage coincided with one of the most tumultuous periods of contemporary Thai politics: it featured seven governments, five general elections, and one coup as entrenched anti-democratic royalist elites and the military opposed the rise of electoral politics. The politically and emotionally charged battles over political legitimacy have impacted how universal coverage is experienced in Thailand. To understand how this new form of state care has altered the Thai political landscape, we need to historically contextualize this shift within the country's experience of developmental modernity, democracy, and neoliberalism.

In modern Thai history, consideration of the population's health as a social and political goal leads back to attempts to construe the legitimacy of state power. The emergence of Western biomedicine and hospital infrastructure in Thailand had explicit implications for the reconfiguration of the Thai monarchy in the early twentieth century. The old regime managed to refashion itself into a modern monarchy partly by promoting biomedicine

(Bamber 1997; Irvine 1982). Prominent medical institutions and public health charities were initiated by and credited to members of the aristocracy, confirming the monarchy's lingering significance in the construction of modernist developmental projects and state paternalism (Jackson 1999b; Thak Chaloemtiarana 1979). During the postwar years, the military-dominated leadership had continued to harness a paternalistic ideology through rural development, as well as fueling anticommunist agenda and sentiments.[9]

Several public health policies were adopted in the 1950s and 1960s, such as infectious disease control and antimalarial campaigns, the introduction of state subsidy for medical professionals working in rural districts, and a nationwide fertility control program that was initially launched in 1970 (Haggard and Kaufman 2008, 133). In organizing public health services at local levels, government investment in village health stations and district hospitals promulgated by several National Economic and Social Development Plans had been crucial. By 1990, all districts in Thailand had at least one public hospital, and this nation- district health system has become the backbone of Thai primary health care policy (Viroj Tangcharoensathien et al. 2018). Another key development made during the mid-1970s and 1990s was the introduction of different health benefit plans that provide financial protection to three targeted groups: low-income households, public servants, and formal sector workers.

While these institutional expansions have contributed to increase state bureaucratic capacity in health, the distribution of health resources remained largely inequitable in Thailand.[10] Public investment had still been concentrated in urban areas, and the well-off population tended to benefit more from government health spending than did the poor (Kuhonta 2003). Given the unequal income distribution that had been exacerbated during the period of rapid economic growth, the deep and sudden economic downturn that Thailand experienced in 1997–98 brought major challenges to the Thai political structure as well as its health care systems. The economic crisis hit hard among vulnerable social groups, especially informal sector workers and the rural poor (Pasuk Phongpaichit and Baker 2000).

The need to redress serious inequalities in Thai society grew to significant proportions after the Asian economic crisis and created new opportunities for change. The Thai Rak Thai Party, led by the controversial tycoon-turned-politician Thaksin Shinawatra, campaigned on pro-poor reforms and eventually won the 2001 elections by a landslide margin, signaling a new era in Thailand's democracy. Thaksin's government speedily implemented universal health coverage alongside other major elements of the party's platform (Pasuk Phongpaichit and Baker 2009), and their poor-oriented policies eventually became Thaksin's crucial political assets ensuring long-term electoral success for parties associated with him. Such rapid implementation was possible because the design of universal health coverage was long prepared by the network of public health professionals and reformists, and the preexisting district health system offered a solid platform for operating different health plans together.[11] With other sociopolitical changes in the aftermath of the 1997 crisis, the implementation of universal health coverage is regarded as a key example that marked the end of the "developmental social contract" originating from previous authoritarian regimes (Hewison 2005, 323) and a new alignment of political power and electoral politics.

The introduction of universal health coverage indicated a new phase of biopolitics in Thailand in which the state pledged to take responsibility for providing welfare benefits to populations experiencing persistent social and economic inequality. At this juncture, universal coverage forms the part of environment in which the poor have to engage in their struggle to survive, and for numerous health care providers, "Health for all" is not a utopian slogan but an arduous and urgent task to be undertaken.[12] Although medical care is expected to be provided as a public good, in the everyday workings of public hospitals, its distribution requires complex negotiations with economic and existential limits. The ways in which this practical contestation over health is experienced give universal access a particular materiality and meaning.

Elicitation as a Concept

Carefully navigating the divergence between the promise and the reality of universal access, this book is concerned with the actual travail that goes into making care possible as a particular form of public provision. Within the system of universal health care, what does it mean to "care"? Is it possible to construe a health care system not only as a set of legal, financial, and technical means of defining the terms and scope of coverage and benefits but also as a larger obligatory circuit responding to human dependence and vulnerability? How can we identify a wider web of interdependencies that cannot be confined to the workings of biomedicine or biopolitics?

My starting point for answering these questions is to recognize that any exploration of how care becomes possible must consider the relational fields that prompt individuals to respond to the needs of others. The concept of elicitation, which I introduce in this book, acknowledges the affective and material state of *being drawn to* relations of care and spells out how this seemingly passive state can actually be constitutive of a radical mode of being and politics.

By elicitation I mean generative capacities entailed in an embodied presence that can induce responsiveness in others and thus create contacts, linkages, and relations of care. Elicitation characterizes the social encounter and the process of making someone into a caregiver. While expressions such as caregiving and care-receiving denote how care is conceived as a one-way flow from the giver to the taker, elicitation highlights how such movement is triggered by the presence and affect of a being in need of care. Care is not simply that one chooses to give or to receive but rather emerges when "one finds oneself drawn to and finds oneself nurturing and caring for" others (Povinelli 2011, 33). Anthropologist Elizabeth Povinelli underlines this state as crucial to understanding how obligation is formulated not by one's own will or determination but by "a very fragile connection, a sense of an immanent connectivity" (33). Elicitation illuminates the emergent process by which this tenuous but unavoidable bind that is necessary to bring forth the obligation to care is caused to form.

Elicitation as an analytical category helps us understand what configuration of agency is required for care. Our daily practices of care prove that we have a skilled capacity to attend to our own and others' needs, and at the same time this faculty presupposes that we are all in need of help at different times and situations. It is a gray area of human subjectivity between autonomy and dependence that is constitutive of all experience of care. In this sense, care is not only competence but also attests to what philosopher Soran Reader calls the "abject features of human life" (2007, 579). Reader adopts the term "patiency" to illuminate the "silenced and 'othered' passive aspects of personhood" (582). While human agents are "passive, needy, constrained, and dependent as well as active, capable, free, and independent" (Reader 2010, 206), the agential conception of personhood fails to illuminate the very significance of one's ability to receive. To receive, or in Reader's words to be a patient, is not to be helplessly acted upon but to allow or to elicit something to be done. Elicitation is an act of doing and of waiting for something to be done. In this sense, not only the one who is caring but also the one cared for has a vital role to play.

Throughout this book, I will illuminate how people in vulnerable situations elicit relations of care by making implicit demands for recognition and obligation. Despite the variation in and complexity of relations of care in biomedical and other contexts, care happens by way of a shared undertaking: "relations have to be made known" (Strathern 2004, 80). By creatively adopting the Melanesian aesthetics of recognition in the field of biomedicine and medical technology, anthropologist Alice Street shows how people seek to "make themselves visible . . . as particular kinds of bodies or persons in the expectation of eliciting a productive relationship" (2014, 24). Persons, bodies, and diseases are not automatically rendered up as comprehensible and treatable by biomedical knowledge, but people's efforts to "make themselves into an object of another's regard" (2014, 27) are what make a health care system work for them, especially in such a heterogeneous setting as Papua New Guinea. Street's work offers crucial insights into how the elicitation and production of certain forms of personhood are a precondition for biomedical and bureaucratic engagement. In a similar vein, I show in chapter 3 how migrant patients, whose entitlement to health care is not guaranteed, actively take part in a documentation process to make themselves and their children visible within the public health system. The medical staff in Ban Phaet Hospital in turn find much of their authority predicated on being recognized as ideal state officials by their patients, local communities, and upper-level institutions (chapter 1).

While Street largely focuses on techniques of visibility and negotiations between those who see and those who are seen, my own conception of elicitation underlines the fragile but immanent sense of co-presence among the parties involved in care. Building on the premise that care stems out of performative modes of relatedness, I broaden the scope of relatedness to include affective entanglement and show how one's very physical and symbolic presence is compelling and has the capacity to draw others into a relationship of mutual obligation. Universal health coverage signifies citizens' right to access health care, yet in the usual operation of public hospitals, citizenship status itself does not assure that care will be delivered. Rather, only the people who occupy hospital spaces and wait can obtain the health care to which they may be formally entitled. Waiting is a temporal and embodied form of elicitation (chapter 2). Co-presence can also account for the difference between dying and growing: critically ill infants cannot argue for their survival, yet their very presence in the intensive care unit forcefully invokes relations of care that cannot easily be repudiated (chapter 4). The ties of mutuality that one has or wishes to have with one's own kin, neighbors, and even other-than-human beings is fundamentally dependent on the effectiveness of elicitation that makes each party feel and act (chapters 5 and 6). In all these different domains, care happens or fails depending on how well one's presence is seen, heard, felt, imagined, and called upon.

The concept of elicitation thus enables us to understand that care is not limited within a dyadic relationship between a "carer" and a "care recipient" but subsists within a broader assemblage implicating varying relations, life forms, institutions, places, technologies, and forces. In this conception, care challenges the simple division between subjugation and resistance, consent and coercion, and dependency and autonomy. Being in another's care or caring for others never frees one from existing social hierarchies and inequality, but one is never simply dominated by them, either. Instead, care as a process of mutual becoming generates effects in all those coming together in an act of care. Indeed, elicitation makes clear that care involves a certain power over life not in the sense of control and mastery but in the sense of trying and enabling. In what ways, then, might this ontology of care disagree with the ideas of omnipotence and power over life, which are centered in the notion of biopower and sovereignty? The theoretical clue that elicitation offers is that there are different ways of thinking and exercising power over and of life.

Power and Potentialities of Life

During my fieldwork at various health and healing sites throughout Chiang Mai, ranging from clinics to people's homes and shrines to spirits, I realized that there were multiple forms of life affecting one another, whether they take the form of citizens, noncitizens, migrants, villagers, ethnic minorities, the documented, the undocumented, pregnant women, newborn babies, disabled dependents, the living, the dying, or the dead. Some distinctions based on nationality, entitlement, and biological attributes are closely linked to the biopolitical state's apparatuses to demarcate and normalize the population, while others are not. Instead, they correspond to multiple temporalities and vitalities of human life.[13] The dynamic process in which life is born, grows, and debilitates also corresponds to particular relations of nurture, perseverance, control, and mutuality. Being attuned to the manifoldness of life allows us to see the multiplicity of forces operative both within and beyond biopolitics.

Thai and Shan cosmologies of life and power are not exotic cultural backgrounds but rather effective guides to the forcefulness of care and its possible rendering, with allowance for "the animacy of the lifeworld" (Ingold

2011, 68). In Chiang Mai as in many parts of the world, the living and the dead intimately intermingle to make life possible, and both human and nonhuman entities are drawn to relations of care.[14] Here, elicitation matters as a way of grasping how human life might be dependent on various nonhuman entities. Tim Ingold defines animacy as "the dynamic and transformative potential of the entire field of relations within which beings of all kinds, more or less person-like or thing-like, continually and reciprocally bring one another into existence" (2011, 68). Spirits and other sorts of nonhuman entities exist in this relational field, and they exert a certain power. In this field of animated beings, their force may not be actualized, but it is still potent.

Let me bring you back to the ward, where I began, and the 10-baht coin under Lung Bun's hospital bed. It was a small offering to the spirit for staying in Uncle Bun's bed. As Aunt Deng explained to me, "After a person has died on a bed, their *winyan* (spiritual essence) remains there. So we give them money and let them know that we will borrow their bed for a while. And if the spirit wants to take this bed back, it will help the patient to get better soon, so it can stay alone in the bed." That day I found out that among the eighteen beds in the male ward, six had coins hidden away for the spirits. The spirits' power to heal was there ready to be elicited through a ritualistic technology.

The offering to the spirit in the hospital bed encapsulates an indigenous conception of the body and the logic of healing and protection. The human body is a contested site where various forces linger and interact. The vicissitudes of life are associated with the movement of life forces and nonhuman entities.[15] If *khwan* and *winyan* (spiritual essences) are not properly attached to the body, the person can become sick or possessed by nonhuman entities. The permanent departure of spiritual essences from the body would mean death. After death, the *winyan* turns into a *phi* (a spirit, or disembodied supernatural agent). The spirit can cause suffering, illness, and misfortune, or it can provide protection, security, and prosperity. Its ambivalent power can manifest itself as either malevolence or benevolence. More powerful and higher spirits and deities are involved in the affairs of human and nonhuman entities as the lords of life and place.[16]

This conception of the spirit reveals one of the central power dynamics found widely in Thai and Shan cultural traditions and more generally in Southeast Asia. Power is not mere dominance; instead it relates to potency and potentiality. Various life forces are also invested in certain sounds, words, images, objects, and places. In this topology of animacy, it is necessary to elicit these forces to manifest themselves as sources of security, prosperity, nurturance, and well-being.[17] Nicola Tannenbaum's (1995) classic study on Shan Buddhism notes the coupling of power and protection as the main thread of religious tenets and cultural practices in northern Thailand's Theravada world. Here, power is conceived as a passive force that is pulled and pushed through a relational field. Power is attributed not only to certain sacred beings that can ward off danger but also to relatively weak beings, such as lower spirits and humans, which are vulnerable to harm. These lower beings derive power from their capacity to constitute efficacious relationships with sources of protection (Tannenbaum 1995). By carefully glossing Buddhist conceptions of protective powers and potential enlightenment, historian Craig Reynolds also stresses that configuring power in this religious tradition "is not the inherent property of an object or agent but the possibility, the becoming, the not-yet-realized" (2005, 217–18). In this ontology of power, spirits' ability to protect and to harm is not predetermined but is constantly reshaped as it is actualized in practice.

This book proposes that if we look closely at the animated dynamic in which power over life emerges as a passive force or untapped potential, we can gain new insights into a manifestation of state power and its biopolitical formation. Within Southeast Asian studies, a number of scholars have discussed the importance of such cultural concepts of power and have shown how rural political societies and national governments' development projects are built on the ideas of the state as a field of potency and an ambivalent source of abuse and prosperity.[18] Like spirit power, state power can also be malleable and either destructive or nurturing. Then again, the question of how to elicit and reify the state's capacity to care becomes central to people's everyday dealings with governmental agencies. Here, the state provision of welfare and health is not only a technical field of intervention but also something suffused with immanent forms of obligation that are subject to elicitation.

The indigenous logic of power, protection, and healing found in northern Thailand informs the way we rethink care as a form of power that is not based on the notion of acting unilaterally on life but instead emanates from interactions and relations among humans and nonhuman beings. Elicitation may consist of a request in the form of a mere gesture, but it is nevertheless a vital process in the sense that it can be one of "the modalities of interactions between ontologically different beings that life cause to emerge" (Pitrou 2014, 102). Scenes of waiting, nurturing, imagining, and becoming that this book painstakingly depicts allow us to see how the person who is the object of care is not merely the product of power over life but is also a producer that itself gives new life forms to various human and nonhuman agents to become a caregiver.

Care in Place

The stories I tell in this book come from diverse settings and are exploratory in nature. I started my research by learning about the trajectories of certain hospital patients' illnesses and followed their journeys from the hospital to their homes or vice versa. I eventually ended up immersed in a ramifying circuit of paths that connect biomedical and bureaucratic mechanisms, persons, sacred loci, and potent objects. Over time I came to write about unexpected capacities invested in this circuitry of care.

The book begins with the central node of Ban Phaet Hospital and its connecting paths, which provide a layout of the local landscape of Chiang Mai. The first chapter describes the institution's daily cycle and flows of people in and out of it. The workings of the district hospital provide a lens for examining the poor and marginalized populations' reliance on the state provision of health care. As a centralized insurance plan, universal health coverage imposes national standards for eligibility and benefits upon contracted institutions. Yet the staff at Ban Phaet Hospital do not unconditionally conform to these bureaucratic rules but rather rework them to offer the care that they believe their patients need. While potential tendencies of power—care and exclusion—can be entertained in this biopolitical mechanism, the hospital staff aspire to realize what the ideal state is thought to offer: accountability for people in need. In this proposition, the district hospital does not work for the government but rather as a government through the conjunction of caring and governing that characterizes sovereign power over life.

The pressing dilemma that the hospital staff have to face is that although they are willing to provide health care for all, the delivery of care may be delayed due to a lack of resources. In this context, filling in the gap between the ideal and the actual becomes the shared burden of the hospital staff and users. Chapter 2, "Patient Waiting," traces the wide spectrum of affects observable in the hospital, ranging from gratitude to frustration, dissatisfaction, deference, and indebtedness. These affective responses reveal how free health care is experienced as an imbalanced gift or debt. Drawing on people's popular evaluations about the public hospital, especially complaints, gossip, and rumors, shows how the aura of former prime minister Thaksin Shinawatra and the monarchy is evoked with regard to questions of political legitimacy and the obligation it entails. In this intersubjective realm, state aid is not freely allotted but rather carefully elicited within an affective weave of moral dependence and autonomy.

In this vernacularization process of universal access, the question of who constitutes a legitimate subject of care demands greater attention. While the bureaucratic framework of universal health care benefits limits its coverage to legal Thai citizens, in Chiang Mai there are many whose membership in the nation-state is questionable but who seek care and treatment. As a pivotal borderland of mainland Southeast Asia, a key feature of this region is the confluence of multiple ethnicities, including Khon Mueang (northern Thai people), Shan, Karen, Hmong, Akha, and Lisu people and of migrants from neighboring countries. It is a home to a great number of documented and undocumented Shan and Burmese migrants, as the globalized Thai economy has absorbed an influx of disfranchised people escaping military violence in the conflict zones of Myanmar/Burma and seeking economic opportunities.[19] In this context, Ban Phaet Hospital is not in a border area but operates as a front-line health care provider for itinerant workers, ethnic minorities without nationality status, and people without citizenship. Among various impoverished noncitizen inhabitants who cannot but rely on the public provision of health care, Shan migrant women are protagonists who reconfigure the horizon of universal access through artful practices of elicitation.

Focusing on Shan migrant women's predominance in the antenatal clinic, chapter 3, "Careful Inscription," illustrates how the interstice between human and citizen begins to be bridged through the routine of reproductive health services for the unborn and their mothers. Despite migrant women's legally ambiguous status, their active use of antenatal care paves the way for demanding recognition and membership in the local hospital and the state. My interest is in showing how the biopolitical process of verification and documentation brings about an unexpected realm of presence. The cooperation between antenatal nurses and Shan women is an unusual alliance in which noncitizen subjects, alien migrants and their unborn babies, become legitimate and desired subjects of care. Birth documents, the outcomes of collated inscription work, prove that these noncitizen subjects are anchored in the realm of state protection.

Newly born human beings also embody the force of elicitation. In chapter 4, "Premature Life and Death," I look at how intensive care is organized for critically sick infants. Responding to the chronic shortage of neonatal intensive beds in Chiang Mai, Ban Phaet Hospital began to offer treatment to newborns regardless of their or their parents' citizenship status. Within the liminal threshold between birth and life, sick and premature newborns' utter dependence on life-sustaining care brings us an unusual manifestation of power over life. By tracing medical staff's efforts to be accountable to their extremely vulnerable patients, I show that withdrawing intensive care—and letting patients die—is also relational work that requires affective involvement and distancing through commensality, prosthetic extensions, and karmic network. This specific mode of care, which is premised on a combination of unconditional openness and careful detachment, offers crucial insight into care as an enactment of hospitality.

Shan women's experience of pregnancy and child-rearing pushes us to contemplate the deeply troubling toil of care undertaken by marginalized migrant women. Chapter 5, "Struggles at Home: Nurturance and Vulnerability," recounts the risk, danger, suffering, and hope embedded in gendered work for the self and family. Paying close attention to Shan mothers' struggles in the milieu of economic scarcity and violence, it shows how the dual weight of child-rearing and wage labor threatens these women's own health and basic security. In their struggle, enacting the maternal role takes divergent forms as they adopted the different methods of elicitation. These women's struggle to take care of their own bodies and souls as well as of their young children and family reveals the small but significant moments of everyday life in which home turns out to be an experimental place where possibilities for transformation, healing, and betterment happen.

The question of how different forms of life interact with each other is further explored in chapter 6, "Spirits and the Circuitry of Care." In this chapter, I consider how the availability of deities occurs through local circuits of care connecting the hospital to the patients' homes and the shrines of spirit mediums. Mediums' and their devotees' narratives and ritual technologies allow us to grasp how spirits come to have significance in maintaining and enhancing human life. By delving into afflicted families' attempt to invoke spirits' protective power, I suggest that the everyday genre of devotion hints at the imaginative aspects of eliciting care. Care is imaginative practice not in the sense that spirits are not real but in the sense that their presence has to be enacted by creative speculations. The provisional but tangible alliance between humans and spirits offers an evidence of care as a potentializing force that is dependent upon the contingency and fragility of life.

Finally, the concluding chapter brings together various ways in which care is compelled and emanated in the previous chapters and discusses the significance elicitation can have in a broader politics of distribution. Care may not be the most effortless means to overturn the dominant political orders that dispossess us, but it is nevertheless a powerful act as it amplifies the presence of life in many forms, provokes tensions, and augments moments of responsiveness.

~

One of the strengths of this book is that it allows us to envision the landscape of care by tracing and tracking people's lives and biographies; however, in doing so, problems are encountered with regard to translation and communication. Northern Thailand is a multilingual and multiethnic place, and many of its residents made efforts to switch from Northern Thai to Central Thai, and also from Shan to Northern Thai, in order to communicate with me.[20] I received much help in learning and understanding these languages from nurses, doctors, and my foster family members with whom I lived during my fieldwork. I was also aided by several brilliant student collaborators from Chiang Mai University. I conducted most of the interviews myself but received help from Shan research collaborators who speak English for the interviews with newly arrived migrants who spoke little Northern Thai.

My imperfect translations have undoubtedly led to a loss in meaning in some cases. During my fieldwork, I sometimes understood only bits and pieces of events and was compelled to wait for some stories to be retold, disseminated, and reexplained. Especially in hospital settings, my main methodology was being present, and the most of time I had to wait until medical staff, patients, or their relatives had the time to explain what had happened, all the while diligently taking notes on what I saw and heard. The conversations I quote in this book are the results of repeated revisitations of words and phrases. Through this chain of retelling and retracing, unknown things were partly but sometimes compellingly revealed, and I could be connected to the lives of the people who told me their stories. Storytelling allowed me to coordinate and assemble meanings within the uncertainty and instability of translation.

Ethnographic stories are indeed a means for producing situated knowledge. I began my fieldwork for this project in 2010, eight years after the nationwide adoption of universal health coverage (UHC), at the point that the institutional and legislative changes introduced at the center had been fully implemented on the local level while the pre-UHC time still remained in public memory. I conducted eighteen months of intensive fieldwork between 2010 and 2012—years of deep political polarization in Thai society and the immediate aftermath of those years—and returned to Thailand in 2014, 2015, and 2016 for follow-up visits and to observe how this reform has effected irreversible changes in the relationship between the state and the poorest segments of the population.

At the early stages of my research, I intended to work at the district level, where I could grasp the relationship between local communities and the hospital. I visited a total of fourteen district hospitals in semiurban and rural areas in search of a field site. Ban Phaet was ideal in terms of its location and size, and more importantly, a senior nurse who had worked in the hospital for more than twenty years showed an interest in my research, introduced me to the hospital director, and helped me settle in the nearby village. I later found that the hospital's morale concerning equal access was particularly high. The fact that the hospital permitted me to conduct research and allowed me access to all aspects of their activities perhaps already proved their confidence in their work. Throughout the book, I have kept the focus tightly on the lived experiences of those whom I met from Ban Phaet Hospital and its neighborhoods, albeit with an awareness that this focus provides only a partial picture of the complex landscape of public health care. In charting this institution's own successes and failures, my aim is not to present it as a representative sample of the Thai health care system but to illuminate both the singularity of the place and the common logic that makes this particular constitution of care possible. In an effort to mitigate any possible adverse effects, I have changed all names of people and institutions and modified identifying details.

Telling the stories of people's struggles to provide and seek the best care possible is an interpretive and political choice that I make in this book. I present how very different kinds of entities—the state, hospitals, doctors, nurses, mothers and fathers, aliens, and spirits—are mutually implicated in the life-sustaining web of care. In each of the chapters, I demonstrate how the everyday scenes of healing, nurturing, and governing are populated by these entities and illuminate their work of fixing problems, desiring, adopting, improvising, forming and severing connections, and making life matter. My goal in this ethnography is to capture this dynamic and formative potential of care.

I

The Government of Care

The District Hospital

From the historic central market of Chiang Mai one can take a minibus to get to Ban Phaet Hospital. There are two bus routes: the old one crosses the Ping River and the highway that rings the city, traveling along a narrow two-lane road through rice-farming villages, small markets, and old subdistrict centers. The new road, the faster way, passes through somewhat different scenery on the outskirts of the city: a drive-through McDonald's, a fancy supermarket chain selling imported goods from Japan and South Korea, garden restaurants, kindergartens teaching only in English, mushrooming construction sites full of migrant workers from Myanmar, and newly constructed condominiums. Scattered along each side of the four-lane highway are these features of the expanding suburbs of Chiang Mai. The two roads eventually meet at the center of the rural district. After passing the lively fresh food market and municipality office (*thetsaban*) and pulling off the road at the intersection with Route 1001, which leads to the northern part of Chiang Mai, one immediately feels the serenity and quietude of the surroundings. From the side of the road a dirt footpath leads to the hospital.

Ban Phaet Hospital is located in a borderland between the city and the countryside. The changes in the geography of Chiang Mai City and the surrounding villages reflect recent socioeconomic transformations in that the conventional urban-rural divide gets blurred in contemporary Thailand.[1] The area surrounding the hospital is unmistakably rural, but the hospital is just twenty-five kilometers away from the city. In the traditional rice-farming villages around the hospital, people call themselves *khon bannohk* (villagers), yet many people in the area take the new road on a daily basis to get to school, work, and the shops in the suburbs. With this effective link, the town's semiurban periphery brings the rich and the poor, old inhabitants and newcomers together.

In this locale, Ban Phaet District Hospital is a destination for local people who seek medical care provided by the government. As the close proximity to the city hints, people in this area have many choices for seeking biomedical care. One can go to clinics and private hospitals—there are several "international" hospitals that offer an interpreter for foreign patients and many private clinics with air-conditioning and even doormen. The choice is wide open to those who can afford the different options. One's ability to pay, type of employment, attitude toward modern and urban lifestyles, perceptions of the public and private health care systems, and condition and urgency of the illness can all affect the choice of where to seek medical care. Nonetheless, as the busy crowd in the district hospital shows, the majority of people in the local area rely on the government provision of public health care.

Old farmers in a nearby village who remember the small house on stilts where formerly the area's only doctor resided have much to tell about the overall development of the hospital and the village. Now, even small roads in the village are paved, the garbage truck organized by the subdistrict office comes once a week, and the health station has turned into a two-story concrete building with inpatient wards. What was once a small health station in the late 1980s has become a sixty-bed district hospital with an emergency room, three ambulances, and even a neonatal intensive care unit. The size of the medical staff has also increased from one physician in 1990 to eight physicians, one dentist, five pharmacists, and fifty-three nurses in 2012. In two decades, the Thai public health care system has achieved remarkable development, to which the history of this small government hospital attests.

One of the leaps was the national implementation of universal health coverage in 2002: this government-funded plan has provided a comprehensive benefit package to previously uninsured populations and has ensured increased access to health care for the poor. It now includes a wide range of outpatient and inpatient services, including chemotherapy for cancer, heart surgery, and drugs for mental illness.[2] With respect to accessibility, the role of the district hospital in rural areas is critical to the success of this new plan because most of the poor population receiving universal health coverage lives in rural areas.[3]

By 2012, Ban Phaet Hospital was providing a full range of primary health care to around 114,000 people in the district. Twelve subdistricts and 126 villages are served by this sixty-bed hospital, and thirteen primary health care units at the village level are under its supervision. The Thai public health sector is subdivided according to regional administration: each district has a district hospital for primary health care, and at the provincial level there are provincial hospitals and university hospitals for secondary and tertiary care. Within this structure, the district hospital is an intermediary institution between the national public health ministry and the local community. While full geographical range of universal coverage has become possible because of the district health system, it has also proved to be a crucial part of the Thai geometry of state administration. Along with the district office, police station, and post office, the district hospital has constituted the apparatus of local government.

Despite the large population it serves, the district hospital is humble in appearance. On very rare occasions young part-time doctors park their Mercedes-Benzes in the hospital parking lot, but the driveway to the hospital is usually crowded with scooters and old pickup trucks. On the concrete post of the back gate, the phone number of Uncle Nung, a *tuktuk* driver, is scribbled for people who need transportation. A few shabby shops around the hospital sell take-out food and everyday goods, and there is a small outdoor noodle shop famous for its blood mixed soup. Vendors are scattered around the hospital's front gate welcoming the flow of people to the hospital and providing sustenance: a grilled pork stall for the breakfast crowd, a coconut ice cream pushcart vendor for afternoon visitors, and Aunt Tui's fried fish ball stand for night shift nurses and late visitors. The hospital has a two-story concrete building for inpatient wards, an outpatient clinic, a delivery room, an ER, and a pharmacy. Another single-story building houses a dental clinic, physical therapy clinic, and consultation room for psychiatric patients. There is another small building for the kitchen and laundry and a residential area for hospital staff. The residential area is separated from the hospital space by a small garden with a well-decorated shrine for guardian spirits (*jao thi*).

The ebb and flow of people changes through the daily cycle of the hospital. At seven o'clock, patients start to flow into the outpatient department, and nurse's aides are busy checking patients' temperature and blood pressure. At 8 a.m., the waiting hall is already full and no empty chairs are left. To fill the waiting time, nurses demonstrate stretches to be done to music. Following the nurses' lead in the exercises are young mothers with crying babies, farmers wearing shorts and flip-flops, young Shan couples, old people leaning on their walking canes, and boys and girls skipping school for dental examinations. By the time the music ends, the doctors have arrived in their consultation rooms and started the morning rounds in the wards; usually four to five general practitioners deal with around three hundred outpatients per day. Their busy day starts with the crowd of people in the waiting hall, briefly pauses in the late afternoon when the outpatient department is closed, and ends with another long waiting line that forms in the small emergency room until midnight. Paramedics bring car accident victims to the small ER. Some nights people die there before they have a chance to be transferred to the provincial hospital. And some nights, drunken men roam the hospital parking lot and expectant fathers wait all night in front of the delivery room.

~

The relentless daily cycle and the constant flow of people prove the vitality of Ban Phaet Hospital, on the outskirts of Chiang Mai City. In this chapter, I bring into focus how the norm of government is situated in this place. The hospital is an archetypal site of surveillance, discipline, and regulation, where medicine is imagined as a possible mechanism for governing populations (Foucault 1973, 1978). While the Foucauldian concept of governmentality helps us grasp biomedical institutions as a crucial site of power, recent medical anthropology has acutely observed the very instability of the grid of biopower (Livingston 2012; Mattingly 2010; Street 2014). Various governmental initiatives are concentrated in the hospital space, yet in the everyday workings of the hospital, their instabilities, fragilities, and fractures—rather than their efficacies—loom large. Indeed, the district hospital is not just a generic part of governmental system but has its own distinctive set of knowledge, objects, functions, and ways of doing things (Mol 2002, 2008).[4] Ban Phaet Hospital, like many other medical infrastructures in poor parts of the world, is neither a site of complete dysfunction nor an exemplary model of high-tech biomedicine. Within its own limits and capacities, this modest district hospital establishes an unsettled trajectory of power over life.

In the pages ahead, I will show how the government of care takes shape on the ground. Here, I use the term "government" in a broad sense that denotes "the set of procedures established and actions conducted in order to manage, regulate, and support the existence of human beings" (Fassin 2012, 1). Ban Phaet Hospital is a local unit of state administration, but it also exceeds its given function by consolidating its own institutional desire to govern and to care. The institutional ethos that Ban Phaet Hospital has cultivated allows us to explore how the normative dimensions of the state and medicine are combined within the hospital staff's everyday practices. As hospital staff try to materialize a particular vision of government, it is not simply a matter of applying disciplinary and calculative measures to the population as a quantifiable object of improvement and intervention (Foucault 2000, 208). Within the hospital, a different set of ideas and practices informs governmental responsibility: responding to vulnerable lives at stake, sustaining and extending care instead of optimizing and economizing it, appears as its means of effectuating the obligation of government. Beginning with the crowded and underresourced ward, listening to the hospital director's ambitions for the institution and accompanying nurses on trips to villages, I look into how intentions and practices of care exert an organizing force that enacts a particular form of government.

The General Ward: "Keep on Caring!"

It was four o'clock one afternoon in June 2012 in the general male ward. The unair-conditioned ward was full of patients, as usual: three nurses and two nurses' aides were busy looking after twenty-four beds in the general ward and four single rooms. I was standing next to bed no. 6, talking with my village neighbors who were visiting their aunt. In bed no. 6, a seventy-two-year-old grandmother, a Thai senior citizen and chronic obstructive pulmonary disease (COPD) patient, was twirling a nasal oxygen tube that she had to wear twenty-four hours a day.[5] During the morning rounds, the doctor, who suspected lung cancer, recommended a transfer, yet her daughter and other family members were not willing to move her to the provincial hospital for advanced care because of the cost of travel. The family did not expect that surgery or chemotherapy would make any difference. "This ward is our second home," the grandmother's daughter told me with a grin. "We can come here anytime, even at midnight, if her shortness of breath gets worse. All the nurses and doctors know our family very well. How lucky we are." The ailing grandmother had been a frequent visitor of the ward, and owing to the benefit of universal health coverage, the family did not have to worry about hospital bills for her repeated and prolonged hospitalizations.

Opposite bed no. 6, Uncle Kae, a forty-two-year-old Shan migrant father, was surrounded by his toddler daughter and wife. Uncle Kae was very weak and greeted me with his eyes only. A day earlier he had been diagnosed as having malignant hepatoma. He had just returned to this ward with a referral letter from the provincial hospital recommending palliative care as an end-stage cancer patient. He could barely drink orange juice with a straw, but his relatives and neighbors came to see him with heaps of food.

I had followed Uncle Kae's treatment trajectory with help from his family members and ward nurses. His family said that Uncle Kae had not been working for five months and complained of severe abdominal pain and weakness. He went only to Ban Phaet Hospital to seek treatment, never to any other clinic or traditional healers. According to his outpatient visit record, he had been to the hospital five times in one month reporting stomach pain, but no one had detected his severe condition, and they had just prescribed him analgesics and gastric ulcer medication. At his last outpatient visit he had a blood test done, and that time the doctor suspected hepatitis and gave him medication for fifteen days. Without improvement, he returned, and at this time he was hospitalized and referred to a specialist at the provincial hospital. A week later, he then was sent back to Ban Phaet Hospital. The doctor in charge of the inpatient ward, rechecking the referral letter from the provincial hospital, explained to me that the reason that the provincial hospital did not offer chemotherapy was because of the size of the cancer in his liver.

In the next row of beds, I could see Jo, a half-paralyzed five-year-old Shan boy, tossing and turning. On the way back from a family trip to a waterfall, their motorbike had been hit by a car. His father, who had been driving, was not injured, and his mother, who had been holding him on the back seat, suffered a broken leg, but the boy had sustained a severe head injury. Unlike Uncle Kae, who was a documented migrant worker covered by the Compulsory Migrant Health Insurance (CMHI), Jo's whole family was undocumented and uninsured.[6] Jo had spent a month in the pediatric intensive care unit in the provincial hospital, and after his condition had stabilized, he was transferred to this ward for recovery. Jo's mother, who wore a cast on her right leg, had slept in the same bed with the boy for twenty days and still did not know how much she owed. No one had mentioned the hospital bill yet, and medical care was still ongoing.

Bed no. 1 held Uncle Ming, a seventy-year-old Thai man with no address or ID number who was not exactly a patient anymore yet remained in the ward. Uncle Ming's infection had cleared up several weeks earlier, but he had nowhere to go. His family had abandoned him some years ago, and the temple he used to stay at had refused to accept his return. So the nurses had to continue writing nursing notes for him, even though he no longer had a disease that needed to be treated. One nurse told me, "We contacted some charities for the elderly, but still could not find any place to send him. So, what can we do? We just keep on caring [*dulae toh pai*]."

The nurse's insistence upon continuing care speaks of both the capacity and incapacity of this ward. On the one hand, its staff was not sufficient to deal with daily patient care without help from the patients' family members. On that day, nurses cared for eight patients each.[7] While they were swamped with paperwork and ward routines, two nurse's aides were also busy filling water jars, changing bed sheets, and responding to all kinds of requests from the patients and nurses. Without a doubt, in this ward the intention to "keep on caring" does not mean that perfect care was delivered. One night no one remembered to change Uncle Ming's diaper, and he had to sleep on a soiled bed. On the other hand, the ward staff are also aware that feeding, bathing, delivering oxygen and basic pain-relief treatment, and providing a place to stay are simple forms of care that are unlikely to bring about drastic improvements. Yet when other technologically advanced interventions were not available, these crude forms of nursing and tending were necessary, despite their limitations. Simply continuing this basic level of care is an insufficient but realistic way to deal with the difficult economic and social realities that typify the ward.

Universal Access and the Poor

As an insurance plan, universal health coverage is based on the legally defined scope of eligibility and the list of provisions.[8] Section 5 of National Health Security Act that establishes the Thai Universal Coverage Scheme (UCS) declares that "the Thai population shall be entitled to a health service with such standards and efficiency as prescribed in this Act." As this legal foundation has universalized health-related social rights, not everyone has been granted the same status and rights as a part of "the Thai population" because in its implementation process the eligibility criteria for universal health coverage was defined along the lines of citizenship.[9] While Thai citizens who were not covered by the Civil Servant Medical Benefit Scheme or Social Health Insurance for private employees were all incorporated within the new single plan, a large number of ethnic minorities who did not have Thai nationality had become excluded from UCS membership.[10] In addition, the health insurance programs for migrant workers and their dependents have been adopted since 2001, but in reality a vast number of them are undocumented and left uninsured.[11] In this context, the duty of care emphasized in the ward is closely connected to the particular ways in which the ideal of universal access to health care is applied in Ban Phaet Hospital.

As this ward deals with management of chronic disease, palliative care for terminal cancer patients, basic trauma care, and providing shelter and food to the abandoned, I was often struck by how little the ward staff took eligibility issues into account in its everyday organization. When I asked about a patient's health insurance status, the nurses and doctors often responded, "I don't know. He is not Thai, so maybe he has a migrant health card? I can check the chart, if you want." Otherwise, the typical answer emphasized the principle of equal care: "It doesn't really matter whether the patient has insurance or not. The government hospital should provide care for everyone."

These common responses are significant for understanding how this institution redefines eligible subjects of universal health coverage. Here it is important to note that the emphasis on equal access does not mean that a sick person's health insurance status is irrelevant in the everyday workings of the hospital. The hospital budget mainly relies on reimbursements from the National Health Security Office (NHSO), a national body for the management and coordination of Universal Health Coverage, and within this budgetary structure the health insurance status of each patient is carefully recorded and systemically managed through the patient's chart, the computer network, and regular internal audits. The hospital staff also know well that services and treatment given to uninsured patients, mostly non-Thai citizens, are not reimbursed by the NHSO and usually result in financial losses for the hospital.[12] This financial aspect of health insurance is undoubtedly a concern for hospital staff, but in this institution it does not constitute a definitive reason to deny care to uninsured patients.

Instead, the scope of the government hospital is seen as extending beyond the issue of insurance coverage. When I asked the head nurse of the ward about her plans for uninsured long-term patients, she explained, "There is nothing we can do. We have to continue care until they get better and are ready to go home. This hospital belongs to the government. We cannot ask people to pay." A junior nurse who overheard my question to the head nurse joined the conversation and succinctly summarized the character of the patients she had taken care of: "How on earth can these people pay their bill? Look at them. They are dirt poor [*jon ja tai*]." The continued care for these patients in the district hospital is perceived as an obligatory extension of the government's responsibility toward the poor.

Although universal health coverage is a historical product of the shifting paradigm of state health provision from targeting the poor to universal access, the unchanged reality that Ban Phaet Hospital staff have dealt with is that this local government hospital is most likely to be a last resort for the poor who have no other choice. Within the logic of insurance, noncitizens' access to health care can and should be denied, yet the ward is often full of documented and undocumented migrants, ethnic minorities without Thai citizenship, those who have been abandoned, and ailing chronic patients. And for the hospital staff, the working protocol for dealing with this situation is helping the poor. Instead of distinguishing patients into eligible and ineligible groups based on their individual coverage, they are inclined to consider all of them who are present in the ward as legitimate and deserving subjects of care.

When the obligation of government to care takes priority over the transactional aspects of health care service, it is less a function of medical staff's compassion for the poor than it is the result of their shared sense of public service. I began to realize that there is a vernacular political philosophy of government that animates this institutional ethos of care. Among many enthusiasts of this line of thinking is Dr. Kiat, the director of Ban Phaet Hospital, who actively deploys the norms of government in the hospital. I therefore turn now to his office.

The Hospital Director's Office: "We Are the Government!"

Dr. Kiat, a physician in his fifties with an MBA, has confined his career path to public health, unlike many of his college classmates, who have become successful in the private sector. Highly respected for his enthusiasm and dedication to the development of rural hospitals, he often goes beyond the normal duties of a hospital director, consulting with outpatients early in the morning to shorten patients' waiting time. On one day, after his morning consultations ended, we had a long conversation in his office about his career trajectory and the importance of universal health coverage. At one point I mentioned some American health care horror stories from Michael Moore's documentary *Sicko*—dumping patients who could not afford the hospital bill in the street—as an example of the perils of health privatization. He instantly responded, "That's a place we can call a living hell, right?" He then continued to emphasize his and the hospital's duty to provide care: "Health care is a right, not a commodity. That's why the American system is so terrible. If one wants to be rich, they should become a businessman, not a doctor. Being a doctor is not in any way related to being rich and successful. The priority of medicine is saving human life and taking care of the local community. Not making money."

His reasoning about the operation of a government hospital came at a significant moment because at that time his discussions with me also made clear the growing financial deficit of the hospital: as the proportion of uninsured patients increased, it became a financial burden for the hospital. When I mentioned the chronic budgetary issues of public hospitals in Chiang Mai, where the size of uninsured populations was huge, his response was clear.[13] "It doesn't really matter whether the hospital has a financial loss or not. If you can continue to provide service, then the budget eventually will arrive. As a public hospital, we shouldn't worry about making money. Whether the patient has a card or not shouldn't be the concern of medical staff. It's only a concern for the NHSO (National Health Security Office) that wants to play with the budget. But the public hospital does not have to follow the NHSO rules all the time. We are the government [*ratthaban*] here, and it means we should provide care for everyone."

The hospital director offered not so much a generalized position on the human right to health as a confirmation of the hospital's position on its moral duty as a governmental institution. In his claim, health care is a moral and political virtue that demonstrates in a sense that providing care is a way of enacting the potentialities of government. According to his personal conviction, the district hospital is not the bottom of the public health structure, accepting orders from the higher-level state administration, but rather a governing entity that is largely autonomous. When the duty of government and the normative character of medicine become closely connected with one another, it is the desire to care that becomes central to the workings of the government hospital.

It took me quite some time to understand the desire for self-realization that Dr Kiat and several other nurses and doctors shared. The overlap between the moral commitment to saving life and working as a government was more clearly addressed through the hospital director's own struggle to set up the neonatal intensive care unit (NICU) in Ban Phaet Hospital. As an attempt to solve the chronic referral problems for newborn patients in Chiang Mai, he initiated fundraising by asking for contributions from other rural hospitals, and in 2006 Ban Phaet Hospital finally opened the NICU, equipped with four incubators.[14] "Back in the day, we even had to send our infant patients to Nakhon Sawan. Do you know where Nakhon Sawan is? It's just four hours away from Bangkok by car. Because there were no beds left for them in Chiang Mai, we had to go that far away. What nonsense. Chiang Mai University Hospital's NICU was too small to handle the large number of premature babies in this region. We needed an extra neonatal ward, so I proposed the plan to launch a new NICU in my hospital. The Ministry of Public Health was not supportive at all at the beginning. Lots of people laughed about our plan to launch a NICU in this small hospital. But we could not just sit on our hands and watch when babies were dying in the ambulance because there was no place for them."

When the director told me of his struggles to set up the NICU at the district hospital level—although at the beginning it was more like a neonate nursery—I was curious to hear how a sense of shame became a mobilizing impetus: "Before we set ourselves up, no one tried to help us. We had to start on our own. People at a higher level, the Ministry of Public Health or the National Health Security Office, might not feel any shame at the fact that we couldn't save those babies' lives at that time. They didn't think of it as their responsibility. Chiang Mai is the second largest province in Thailand, but we didn't have enough beds left for sick newborns. They didn't feel these things. They just watch us. That's the thing that they do well. But we know why the NICU is so necessary. Because we take care of people here." Then I asked about budgetary issues for intensive care and the burden of bureaucratic processes in dealing with the NHSO for insurance claims. He answered, "Money issues should not bother the practices of doctors in here. The NHSO only deals with the allocation of the budget. They don't have any power to order us what to do or not. They [the NHSO] are not a government department like the Ministry of Public Health. We are the government [*ratthaban*] who work for the people."

How does this emotive obligation interact with the ideal role of the state? When the division between "us and them," the district hospital and the higher levels of government, is contrasted, the accountability of the state is not taken for granted but has to be achieved by the active aspiration and endeavors of the district hospital. Despite the failure of higher governmental bodies to appreciate the urgency of life-and-death care issues at the local level, the director and several other medical staff share a belief that the district hospital should take action as an arm of the government. In this unfolding, it is crucial to note that the hospital director and nurses do not conceptualize the government as an ordering force above and beyond the hospital. On the contrary, the government and the hospital seem to inhabit each other: governing, the work of government, cannot be realized without their work of caregiving. Through its moral and political act of caregiving, the hospital brings into the relations between the government, human life, and the local population its own distinctive ways of instantiating and exercising state authority, actively engaging in the management of life.

A Day Trip to the Village: Acting Like a Government on the Edge

In attempting to act like the government, Ban Phaet Hospital not only takes on the noble cause of saving lives but also engages in organized efforts to establish a relationship between the hospital and the local population. In developing ties between the hospital and the local community, the nurses take on an especially pivotal role. Whereas physicians' work is generally confined within the hospital, nurses' duties often go beyond the boundaries of the ward and hospital. Engaging with the local people (*chaoban*) and community (*chumchon*) is what many of the nurses positively embrace as their own area of work. Nurse Ubon, a fifty-two-year-old woman who has been working in Ban Phaet Hospital for twenty years, once told me of her pride as a nurse: "I hope that my daughter also becomes a nurse. It's a good job that allows you to help less fortunate people and make merit. . . . Our job is taking care of the patient as a nurse and as a public servant as well. [These two roles] cannot be divided. Our work is for the patient, for the region, and for the nation. It covers all. And we work for ourselves too. This job gives us money to live, right? So we work for ourselves, for the patient, and for *ratthaban* [the government]. That's our job as nurse." This kind of account is commonly related by senior nurses who rank as public servants.[15]

This dual duty of state nurses became clearer after I accompanied nurses several times on their visits to patients' homes. Nurses in Ban Phaet Hospital voluntarily organize several "field trips" to visit patients: these home visits are mostly for first-time mothers, COPD (chronic obstructive pulmonary disease) and PD (peritoneal dialysis) home care patients, and bedridden elderly patients. The senior nurses in the inpatient ward and outpatient department make their own lists of patients for home visits, usually those who have been hospitalized repeatedly or who "have complex problems." Thai as well as Shan young mothers receive visits regardless of their health insurance status. Once the home visit schedule is set up, the senior nurses invite other nurses and nurses' aides to join in on these trips. When the nurses arrive in a village, they usually stop at the village health station, and local health volunteers join them in helping find a patient's house. In this process, the impetus of the home visit comes from the senior nurses. There are no direct instructions from the hospital director or the upper-level administration for this type of community outreach. Normally the senior nurses assess the workload in the ward and outpatient department and find time for home visits.

By tagging along on the nurses' trip to see impoverished families in the local villages, old shacks on remote fruit farms, and provisional camps for Shan migrants behind the golf course, I was gradually introduced to the familiar and unfamiliar neighborhoods around the hospital. For their visits, the nurses did not set exact appointment times, but in most cases, families were at home and occasionally prepared cold drinks and homegrown fruit for the guests. Patients and their families addressed nurses using the word for doctor (*moh*) out of respect, although they clearly knew the difference between the professions. The nurses brought a basic medical kit, but the main purpose of their visit was not really to provide medical treatment. The nurses mostly spent their time looking around the house, sitting together with the patients and their families, and having brief conversations. By doing this, and through direct and indirect questions and observations, they tried to learn more about the patients' living conditions, including the state of bedridden patients' beds, ventilation, basic hygiene, and adherence to medication regimes.

While the core aim of these home visits was to help the nurses understand their patients' condition more concretely, this desire to know did not necessarily lead to interventions. In some cases, the family or neighborhood problems were too great for them to solve: the house was literally falling down, the main caregiver of the family was burned-out and neglected the patient for that reason, or in the cases of some migrant mothers, not only their newly born but other sick children also needed help. In these situations, the nurses were sympathetic but also stuck firmly to the original purpose of the visits and avoided intervening in family and neighborhood issues, given their limited resources. What was notable about this kind of community outreach was that it enabled the nurses to learn about their patients and have a significance in the local community.

Nurse Phim, a senior nurse in the outpatient department who was also in charge of the community management of high blood pressure patients, often invited me along on her home visits and updated me about the prognosis of the patients we met together. She remarked, "It's important to let the patients and their family know that we are concerned about them. We try to give them *kamlang jai* [emotional support] so the patients can know that we are interested in them. And so their family can have some strength to take care of the patient." The home visit is not just about how the nurses publicly present themselves to the local community but also about letting people know that they and the hospital care. In addition, the purpose of the home visit was not so much to meet the needs of patients' families as it was to elicit recognition from the community.

In a way, these trips function to extend the medical gaze from the ward into the home, evoking the motifs of regulating and directing the patients' behaviors. Not only clinical examinations in the consulting room but techniques of classifying, locating, and inspecting patients' everyday life also render the kinds of bodies and persons visible and knowable.[16] Yet the interesting consequence of this institutional project is that it has never been a strategic instrument of governing the local population. These visits aim neither an official assessment nor a supervision of the conduct of the family. No specific policy directs the organization of these visits, which are not reported beyond the hospital itself. No system exists for integrating the results of the visits with care plans, and no statistics are generated. Rather, the most evident outcome of this project is that the territory of the district hospital is demarcated by the circular movements of the nurses who were willing to transmit a sense of understanding and support. By organizing home visits, nurses publicly perform an affirmation of the ongoing relationship between the hospital and the patients in the local community. Here, nurses exhibit not only a desire to see their concerned patients but also a desire to be seen by them as a reliable sources of care.

Governing and Caring

This dual desire proves how a particular logic of care infiltrates a microcosm of government. Let us recall the inpatient nurse's remark about *dulae toh pai* (to keep on caring): the verb *dulae* denotes not so much a feeling (caring about) as an action (caring for others).[17] It does not signify indifference to the pain and agony of patients and their families but rather underlines the way that caring manifests itself in situated actions. Caring for others includes a diverse array of possible interactions: examples include maintaining health and safety, providing protection, nourishing, managing, controlling, or restraining.[18] Perhaps most importantly, this concept of care embraces an implicit notion of governing. The *Royal Institute Dictionary* offers an interesting example of the combination of caring and governing. *Pokkhrohng dulae* (to govern and care) is a power attributed to public servants.[19] As Thai grammar requires no conjunction when two verbs are used together, this expression neatly conveys how the jobs of nurse and public servant are enmeshed in the concurrent domain of governing and caring.

This close association between the words "to care" and "to govern" is even reflected in the nurses' uniforms. While the typical image of a white-clad nurse evokes a gendered symbol of compassion and professionalism, nurses in the district hospital have three different uniforms: a white uniform for working in the ward, a blue checked trouser uniform for community outreach, and a military-style government official suit for state rituals. These different outfits for nurses are not so much a reflection of how their duties are compartmentalized as they are an expression of how nurses can conduct distinctive but overlapping projects of caring and governing.

This twofold mode of acting like a government becomes possible because the hospital staff understand, experience, and embody the state as a source of personal and institutional agency. In the anthropology of the state, relationships between state officials and local people have been given great importance as the "critical components through which the state comes to be constructed" (Gupta 1995, 378). Here it is crucial to note that when low-ranking state officials act as a platform for encountering the state at the local level, their daily work is not completely absorbed into the preserve of a monolithic state but contains varying imaginaries and practices that redefine what the government can and should do. The hospital staff are willing to follow all rules of insurance plans and other state prescriptions, but they are not simply following orders. Rather, they expand on the notion of state obligation by setting their goal at having the capacity to protect and care for the people in their charge.

It means that the myriad ways in which public health care is delivered at the district level, then, cannot be entirely collapsed into disciplinary mechanisms and bureaucratic rationalities. The hospital is based on a system of classifications and regulations determined by health insurance and other administrative mechanisms, yet these do not necessarily direct every aspect of hospital management. Rather, an indispensable part of its care practices has to do with the imagined and embedded virtue of the state. At the same time, the obligation to care is not simply a moral disposition solely relying on medical ethics but also a series of institutionalized and bureaucratized projects through which governing the local populations is rendered possible. Within this conception of caring and governing, the two are not contrasting or opposing values but rather concurring modes of work that effectuate potential tendencies of power over life.

What emerges from this concerted practice of caring and governing is perhaps close to what anthropologist Caroline Humphrey (2004) called a "localized form of sovereignty." Rejecting a notion of sovereignty as only a negative assertion of hegemonic power, she calls for a focus on practices, lifeways, and "actualities of relations" to grasp how a local micro-world involves a kind of sovereignty by formulating "its own distinctive ways of instantiating and symbolizing authority, which imposes a specific kind of relationality with its subjects" (2004, 435). The district hospital is conjured up as a micro-sovereign entity when it becomes a center of efficacious networks that engage with the local population. As a state institution, the hospital can exercise its power of constituting a certain group of people as expendable bodies that can be allowed to die in the service of "calculated management of life" (Foucault 1978, 140). Yet, instead of making a "zone of abandonment" (Agamben 1998), Ban Phaet Hospital creates its own zone of caring and governing, by adopting rules of universality that take account of the presence of the people demanding life-sustaining resources and relationships and by making its operational capacity known to patients, local communities, and other state institutions.

Central tensions embedded in this microgovernment of care is that its working is under the influence of larger political processes and that the injunction to "keep caring" runs up against feelings of disappointment, frustration, and uneasiness despite its intention. In the next chapter, we look into how patients and local residents experience and interpret this localized materialization of care, especially within the context of recent Thai political history that is marked by repeated political upheavals and regime changes.

2

Patient Waiting

When Ruen, a patient with end-stage renal failure, stayed in Ban Phaet Hospital, the purpose of his hospitalization was to wait for a chance to be referred to the tertiary hospital that could offer him dialysis. Ruen's income as a landless day laborer meant he could not afford to go to a private hospital, so receiving treatment through universal health coverage was the only remaining hope for him. During the morning rounds, when the doctor asked him how he was doing, Ruen replied with a hint of sarcasm, "I'm still waiting [for the referral]," anticipating the doctor's typical response: "Let's wait for a bit more." During a month-long hospitalization, Ruen told me about his frustration with the futile regime of medication he had been on, yet most of the time he remained quietly in the ward and withheld complaints about his deteriorating condition and the slow response of the public health care system. As he often told me, "I can stand pain, a man should be able to stand pain." However, it was quite obvious that his immensely swollen body was unable to endure much more. He had become delirious and was beginning to lose control of his bodily functions. The ward nurses and doctors were also seriously concerned about the long delay in getting him treatment. Despite their concern, the medical staff also had to wait because they did not have much power to negotiate with specialists at the tertiary level. After numerous contacts, a ward nurse finally arranged an appointment for Ruen with a nephrologist. While no one could anticipate when Ruen would receive dialysis treatment, patience and painful endurance seemed the only course for him as he was utterly dependent on the public health care system.

While Ruen was stuck in the ward with little hope of getting life-saving treatment, his waiting had two effects. On the one hand, it was an active way of holding onto the given situation: as long as he stayed in the ward, the nurses and doctors had to do something for him. On the other hand, waiting—the temporal submission to uncertainty—was an inherently passive and despondent experience: there was nothing Ruen could do about the long delay but wait. The crowded quietness of the ward was symptomatic of how care was dispensed by public hospitals in Thailand. Not only Ruen but also many other poor people in the ward, emergency room, and waiting hall calmly waited their turn to be attended to. A nurse once told me, mixing Thai and English words, "Patients must wait first. Patients *tohng* [must] be patient." What does it mean to be a patient subject who must wait? What are the sociopolitical structures that permit and legitimate the waiting of people who seek help? Which ideas, feelings, and emotions are being expressed and suppressed in this condition of waiting?

In this chapter, I turn to how people who rely on care from public hospitals understand and experience universal health coverage. As both a national and local political process, the establishment of universal health coverage has brought into contentious political debate the meanings of the state, populism, and entitlement in contemporary Thailand. While long waiting times are often regarded as proof of the inefficacy of state-funded public health care, I am more interested in how the promise and failure to provide necessary care form a relational field within which hospital staff, patients, their family members, and the state interact with each other. I open with Ruen's experience to bring attention to how waiting becomes a precondition of accessing public health care. After spending time with Ruen and his family in the ward for many days, I began to recognize that his patient waiting not only spoke to the structural causes of prolonged suffering but also constituted a kind of existential demand for care under conditions of dependence.

Turning from the hospital staff to the hospital visitors, I particularly focus on how universal health coverage is reconfigured as a gift and debt of care, which is situated within intersubjective connections and subject-making processes. I argue that the inner dynamic of universal access found in Ban Phaet Hospital is embodied in sentiments around receiving without reciprocating: a feeling of imbalance continuously structures the ways in which hospital users navigate the treatment process and deal with hospital staff. In this context, waiting is not only a chronic condition of being a recipient of state aid (Auyero 2012); it is also an act that opens up a space for eliciting care. I further suggest that people's embodied practices and concerns over being a proper subject of care denote not only recipients' subordinate position but also their efforts to sustain an obligatory circuit of care and to achieve a sense of mutuality and moral autonomy.

In what follows, I discuss the vernacularization of universal health coverage in Thailand by focusing on the ways in which ousted prime minister Thaksin Shinawatra and the Thai monarchy are invoked as sources of care and social protection. This particular unfolding of universal access shows how providing care for the poor appears as a crucial expression of legitimate power in the contemporary Thai political landscape. I also track down the things people in a dependent situation do, think, and feel while they endure the loops of waiting and powerlessness in their quest to receive health care. A wide spectrum of affects—gratitude, frustration, dissatisfaction, deference, and indebtedness—flowing in the hospital space reflects poor people's insistent efforts to elicit and sustain relations of care.

"30 Baht for Everything!": The Shadow of Thaksin

How do poor Thai citizens who have to rely on public hospitals understand and evaluate the mechanisms of universal health coverage? To answer this question, it is important to know how universal health coverage has been labeled in Thailand. The name on the card that is required for hospital registration is *bat prakan sukkhaphap thuan na* (universal health coverage card), yet people rarely call it this. More often it is called *bat samsip bat* (30-baht card) or *bat thohng* (gold card), using the vernacular names for the official insurance policy. These names denote the per-visit copayment of 30 baht (approximately one US dollar) and the yellow color of the card. But these names also evoke important ideological issues in current Thai politics. After the 2001 election, Thaksin's Thai Rak Thai party accentuated "30-baht health care" as one of their policy highlights. The name *bat thohng* was also used at the launch of the universal health program to emphasize its prestige (Harris 2012, 116) and was again promoted when the 2006 coup regime abolished the 30-baht copayment per visit.[1]

The simple and clear message of *samsip bat raksa thuk rok* (30 baht to treat every disease) is emblematic of the Thaksin government's welfare programs for the poor. During both the rise and fall of Thaksin Shinawatra, universal health coverage was the policy that won most rural voters' hearts.

In 2010, when pro-Thaksin support rallies had reached their peak in his hometown of Chiang Mai, the phrase *samsip bat raksa thuk rok* (30-baht health care) was a regular feature of speeches by local politicians wanting to emphasize the tangible benefits that Thaksin had brought to the people when he was in power.

For many public hospital users, the 30-baht card was a vivid manifestation of Thaksin's presence in their lives. To a seventy-three-year-old Thai woman who had taken care of her husband when he was suffering from stomach cancer, the 30-baht card was the thing she was most grateful to have received through Thaksin's policies. She told me, "Without the card, my husband wouldn't have dared to think about getting cancer surgery." I reminded her that she had mentioned the dreadful waiting times in a provincial hospital: although she and her husband had arrived at the hospital at 6 a.m., they had to wait until the late afternoon. But her response was still firm. She replied, "People who say that the 30-baht card is bad are so stupid. The protection of life is the most important thing. I'm very grateful that Thaksin brought the 30-baht card for the poor, like us. I hope that Thaksin can come back to Thailand soon for us."

This kind of reception shows how universal health coverage has opened a distinctive political space in Thailand. The ways in which universal health coverage (UHC) was labeled as Thaksin's policy effectively turned the structural shift that the introduction of UHC had brought into a personalized political good for a populist politician. The introduction of UHC became possible not because of one man's heroic will but rather as a well-orchestrated outcome of a professional movement. Sociologist Joseph Harris (2015, 2017) has provided a rich account of the coalition movement of public health bureaucrats who created a long-standing alliance between doctors' associations, international agencies, and a political party to pave the way for universal access in Thailand.[2] And the slogan that every condition can be treated for 30 baht has obscured the troubling issues that partly resulted from the rapid launch of universal coverage in Thailand. The problems relating to reimbursement, the public health financing structure, and the rapid expansion of the unregulated private health market were considered during the initial stage of universal coverage, yet these issues were only debated within a very limited circle of bureaucrats, public health experts, and NGOs.[3] For the general public, the policy was presented as an alluring promise of social protection with a hint of a great bargain—a full range of treatments would be offered for only 30 baht.

Yet it is equally important to understand how the popular appeal of this policy, especially among the rural poor, has translated into a populist form of politics.[4] The general popularity of this policy among the rural poor is often used as evidence that this reform is connected to a sheer "populist" plot to lure the votes of the poor majority. But there is much to suggest that the impact of universal health coverage is far more extensive than pork barrel patronage. One statistical study shows that most of the poor Thai population in rural areas has been covered by universal health care and that the poorest quintile of the Thai population has experienced a higher rate of using its services (Supon Limwattananon et al. 2012). Another study also suggests that the current health policy is particularly effective in protecting poor households from health-related financial risks (Tewarit Somkotra and Lagrada 2008). The very sustainability of universal health coverage in Thailand is based on strong support from the poor majority, who have no choice but to rely on state-provided health care; their experience of the state's changing role in providing health care has become fertile ground for electoral politics and political mobilization.

This particular formation of a social policy suggests that Thaksin's political success may have brought about a radical shift in Thai political culture toward a more "direct, universalized relationship between citizen and state" (Pitch Phongsawat 2004, in Pasuk Phongpaichit and Baker 2009, 196). Yet it may be insufficient to define this emergent relationship as a transactional mode of citizenship since universal health coverage appears to have opened up a political field imbued with affective recognition, including a sense of gratitude. In many everyday conversations concerning universal health coverage, it is noticeable that the policy itself often substantiates Thaksin's close attention to the poor. Here I do not argue that rural people simply confuse the political influence of the ousted politician and the role of government in society. Rather, the tales of Thaksin's concern for the poor have become a means by which the relatively complex structure of universal health coverage is made concrete. In people's encounters with the state through health care, Thaksin plays a role as a political symbol, concretizing the state's ability to give care and secure the poor's needs.

The sense of gratitude that characterized the popular response to universal coverage indeed requires a closer look. When the old woman taking care of her husband without any support from her children expressed her appreciation for Thaksin's help, she not only evoked the rural poor's political loyalty to a controversial populist politician but also revealed an affective tie between citizen subjects and the state. As gratitude comes from the acknowledgment of receiving help, what emerges is a form of sociality involving the notion of gift rather than right. Here, people's emphasis on Thaksin's benevolence is not just about their endorsement of his political significance but also about their assertion of the benevolent potential of the state, which is prepared to give care and protection.

The King's Benevolence and Public Health Care

Within the pluricentric sphere of Thai political authority, it is important to note that although Thaksin may be a larger-than-life figure, there is another whose long-standing political aura represents even more strikingly the premise of generosity and care. The modern Thai monarchy has established its position in Thai society as a great source of charity and care by reference to Theravada Buddhist conceptions of kingship.[5] The figure of the selfless king who rules by Buddhist moral law has been carefully crafted through numerous elaborate public demonstrations of the king's generosity and tender attention to his subjects. In particular, King Bhumibol Adulyadej utilized royal charity as a major platform of political influence. Thak Chaloemtiarana (1979, 325–34) notes that the expansion of royal charity reveals how state paternalism has been extended beyond the capacity of the government through the active function of the monarchy. Beginning in the 1960s, royal charity was diversified into disaster relief, donations for anti-communist programs, welfare for the border police and soldiers, development programs for hill tribes, and academic foundations. Paul Handley (2006), the author of King Bhumibol's unauthorized biography, which is banned in Thailand, also extensively tracked down the royal family's strategic involvement in charity and its symbolic and political implications.

Medicine and public health, in particular, have been crucial components in constituting the image of the "development king." The association between the royal family and the introduction of Western medicine started in King Mongut's reign, and it continued with the contribution by Prince Mahidol (the father of King Bhumibol) to the development of modern medical education (Bamber 1997, 243).[6] Based on the records of Privy Council donation lists from 1963 to 1971, Thak Chaloemtiarana (1979, 328) shows that health and medicine were the main objects of royal donations: more than 57 percent of the total donations for this period were granted to hospital medicine and the Red Cross, chaired by the queen. In this systemic and nationwide charity endeavor, it is interesting to note that not only the distribution of money but also gestures of caring and detailed attention have been central to royal charity.

As in other Thai government institutions, the monarchy's image is prominently on display in public hospitals. Not only do hospitals exhibit ceremonial decorations for royal anniversaries and host special rituals commemorating royal charity, but they also use images of the royal family in posters promoting health campaigns around breast feeding, smoking cessation, healthy eating habits, and the like. Given these abundant images of the monarchy, it was not odd to meet people in the hospital space who recalled the monarchy's care and benevolence.

People who evoked the king's generosity in the public hospital were not necessarily anti-Thaksin royalists, but Khaek was a rigorous royalist ready to argue with anyone who spoke up for Thaksin's 30-baht scheme. A fifty-eight-year-old woman who had been working as a cleaner in the hospital for twenty years, Khaek had an uneasy feeling that Thaksin would ruin the people's love for the king.

> The 30 baht [plan] doesn't come from Thaksin. It's all about our tax money. It's so frustrating to hear people saying that Thaksin built the new building of the hospital. That's not true. And these people [Thaksin supporters] don't see how the royal family has contributed to the development of the hospital. Phra Thep ["princess angel," referring to Princess Maha Chakri Sirindhorn] donated all those expensive medical devices, so now the doctors can treat patients, no need to send them to the university hospital. If anything happens like floods, do you hear about Thaksin donating anything anywhere? He is just a greedy businessman. Everywhere the king went he took care of the people and made the place developed. We are so indebted to him [*mi bunkhun yoe mak*]. Thai people see the king's face every day, even on the one-baht coin. If there is a one-baht coin on the ground, I never fail to pick it up, because I'm afraid that people will step on the king's face.

Khaek's emphasis on taxes pointed out the basic financing structure of universal health coverage, yet her argument extended to the monarchy's contribution to public health care. Although she made a clear distinction between the operation of government policy and the Thai monarch, in this narrative public health care and other welfare programs are portrayed as expressions of the king's benevolence. This imagined and felt allegiance between the poor and the compassionate king, or in reverse, the king's obligation to be compassionate to the poor, is deeply rooted in the symbolism of sovereign power and polity.

Regardless of her strong disapproval of Thaksin's political influence, Khaek's narrative shares a similar emotion to that exhibited by Thaksin supporters. *Bunkhun* (debts of merit), a sense of gratitude and indebtedness, touches an emotional and moral register involving the mode of giving and receiving. In its ordinary usage, *bunkhun* often addresses an unconditional or unreturnable gift, such as parents' love for their children. Here, royal donations and charities are fundamental to constituting the meaning of sovereign power in Thailand, not only because the cumulative and systematic propaganda work contributes to the monarchy's ideological domination but also because it identifies the monarchy as a source of care. In this specific way of representation, the king's infinite giving to the poor, and eventually to the nation, is central to his sovereign authority. The affective tie between the sovereign and his subjects is not abstract but is felt immediately and intimately, as Khaek's tender and dutiful reaction to the king's face on the coin suggests.

In stressing that the politics of representing help and expressing gratitude are crucial dimensions of the vernacularization of universal health coverage in Thailand, I am not suggesting a simple equation between the ways Thaksin and the monarchy are implicated in these expressions. Instead, my contention here is that when people's experiences of universal health coverage are shaped by their perceptions of it as the work of government, Thaksin and King Bhumibol come to be known and felt intimately as sources of care. In Thai public health care, gratitude appears as a dominant expression among the poor who have to rely on state health provision, which is largely presented as a sovereign gift. Feeling gratitude might not be the only affective consideration entailed in the process of giving and receiving, yet my argument here is that how and why people hold on to this specific affective tie with state agents needs to be examined closely.

The peculiar features of universal health coverage in Thailand indicate that liberal concepts of social welfare are not sufficient for understanding this relational dimension of state power. Public health care has been rendered as a specific expression of moral and political projects that stem from electoral populism, political paternalism, and residues of bureaucratic pastoral regimes. As universal health coverage has become a way in which the state finds legitimacy in people's lives through giving care, how does the promise of giving provide circumstances for poor people relying on public health care? I use the modality of giving, configured as universal coverage, to gain insights into how this uneasy space of gratitude and indebtedness is experienced.

Waiting and Silent Frustration

A play on the promise of *samsip bat raksa thuk rok* (30 baht to treat every disease) is the joke *samsip bat thuk khon ja tai* (with the 30-baht health plan everyone will die). As this quip suggests, alongside the gratitude of many, one often encounters skepticism about state-provided health care. This is especially true among the middle and upper classes, where the quality of care under the universal health coverage plan is often subject to criticism. Since the 1997 economic crisis, the private health sector has grown rapidly, with the support of the government, and has particularly targeted foreign patients.[7] An important issue posed by the growing private health sector is that universal coverage has turned out to be a program for the poor rather than one alleviating the unequal distribution of health resources between classes.

Waiting is a defining feature of public hospitals, and on any given morning at Ban Phaet, the scene is one of an overwhelming crowd of people waiting. The problem of long waiting times has to do with more than just systemic inefficiency and disorganization. It also raises issues around how people deal with indeterminacy and lack of control. In the space of the public hospital, frustration over waiting and being neglected is ever present. However, among the people who had to rely on public hospitals for necessary care and treatment, there was seldom a word of direct disapproval. The strongest criticism I heard from a family member of a patient was a reference to a *rongphayaban* (hospital) that resembled a *rongkhasat* (slaughter house). He recalled his friend's death from AIDS in the public hospital many years ago: "No one did anything for him. No one cleaned him at all or took care of him. They just put the sick person in the ward and wait till the patient dies."[8] This kind of direct condemnation needs to be explored further with other examples, but in the hospital space, what I began to recognize was how patients and their families became attuned to the condition of waiting.

Rather than voicing their needs or expressing anger at being neglected, most of them accepted that the care and treatment they could get from the hospital always ran up against limits. Within these limits, care often necessitated a posture of calm and patient waiting. "Doing nothing but wait" (*dai tae loh yang diaw*), an expression commonly applied to using the public hospital, underlines not only the discontent of those waiting to receive care but also a principle of navigating the experience. I spent much of my time in the hospital just waiting with my informants in the hallway or in front of the consultation room. Most often people hardly asked the hospital staff how long or why they would have to wait. Gradually, I also came to feel that it was absurd or unthinkable to ask such questions in a busy waiting room packed with other sick people. Here, the waiting that my interlocutors and I readily accepted was not about a calculable duration of time but a habitual way of being in the hospital to receive care.

Based on his long-term ethnographic engagement in poverty and welfare programs in Argentina, sociologist Javier Auyero argues that indeterminate waiting for welfare benefits becomes a "daily lesson in political subordination," and through this "strategy of domination" the urban poor "learn to be patients of the state" (2012, 9). His acute recognition of the banality of waiting as a key characteristic of the interactions between the poor and the state helps us understand how "habitual exposure to long delays molds a particular submissive set of dispositions" (2012, 9). Yet unlike Auyero's emphasis on waiting as a mode of dominance and submission, I direct my concern to the relations between waiting and the obligatory circuit of care. We might recall how public health care has been modified and represented as a kind of gift in the Thai political landscape. Although long waiting in a Thai public hospital commonly involves experiences of the unpredictability and unreliability of a state administration that makes patient-subjects put up with its arbitrary commands, what is prominent in this modality of care is a sense of indebtedness. From the vantage point of giving as an expression of state power, I locate waiting within the deep dilemma of the gift.

In the conclusion of his famous essay on the gift, Marcel Mauss wrote about the link between the ethos of the gift and emerging welfare states. For Mauss, social insurance and the state's "desire to look after the individual" ([1954] 1990, 68) were connected to the reappearance of public giving: at the heart of modern notions of social security, solidarity, and interdependence were old principles of the gift and the obligatory circuit of giving and receiving. The perils of the gift, on the other hand, touch upon another dimension of interdependence associated with unequal power relations: there is a danger that a free gift could wound recipients who cannot reciprocate for what they have received.[9] Like the individuals Auyero observed in the Argentinean welfare office (2012, 122), people in the Thai public hospitals I visited often explained that they were there because they had no other place to go. For people in need, in contrast to people who can choose, receiving free care is paradoxically painful because being on the receiving end of a nonreciprocal act of giving entails the wounding experience of compliance. Waiting, calm waiting in the hospital, is the starting point of being a recipient, a subject of care. In the following, I delve into life in a public hospital, where attempting to pay off the debt after receiving care becomes a serious task for patients and their families.

Kreng Jai: Moments of Uneasy Receiving

Nuwan opened the small sliding window of the nurse station and, politely addressing the nurses inside, said, "The patient said that the pain was too much. Could you come over to see him?" Nuwan's younger brother was an end-stage cancer patient, and at that time his wife and two young daughters were all staying in the ward together. While the other family members could not decide whether it was better to take the patient back home or stay in the Ban Phaet Hospital ward, Nuwan was the only one who tried to discuss her brother's condition further with the hospital staff. As she told me in the corridor, "My sister-in-law said that she feels *kreng jai*, so she couldn't ask the nurses and doctors questions. So they asked me to talk to them. If I didn't ask anything, they would just wait for the nurses to come to the patient." "But don't you feel *kreng jai*?" I asked her. "I used to live in England for twenty years. So my relatives think that I don't act like a Thai anymore," she responded with a grin.

Nuwan is from a family of small farmers. In her early thirties she married a British man and came back to Chiang Mai after her husband died. When her brother was diagnosed with cancer, she began to spend much of her time in several hospitals. The universal health coverage plan covers basic cancer treatment, including chemotherapy, but both the provincial and university hospitals refused to offer any surgery or chemotherapy for Nuwan's brother owing to the size of the tumor. Her brother, who previously worked as a construction middleman, was only thirty-seven years old. After he received a diagnosis but no treatment in the public hospitals, Nuwan took him to a private hospital to ask for a second opinion. A one-day hospital stay and some tests cost Nuwan more than 80,000 baht (USD 2,656). She paid the bill but could not afford any more, so they went back home. When the pain became unbearable, eventually Nuwan's brother returned to the Ban Phaet Hospital ward where he had first been admitted.

Nuwan herself had also received stomach cancer surgery when she was in England. "I lived there for more than ten years and paid tax as other people did. So I paid only 50 percent of the treatment cost. But my husband was English, so he did not have to pay anything when he was sick." "Did you feel *kreng jai* when you were in the hospital in England?" I asked. Nuwan explained to me:

> No, not at all. People in England think that they have a right, because they pay tax for that. But Thai people think that the government hospital provides treatment for free. Some people don't know that they paid their tax already. Rich people go to private hospitals and get whatever special service they want. But people using public hospitals think that it's free, so they should be grateful and [feel] *kreng jai*. It's already good to get free care, so people think that it's better not to ask for more and not to bother the hospital staff. "Just wait for a while, they are all busy. The nurse will come to us later." People say things like this, although they have many questions they want to ask. All of my relatives feel uncomfortable to call on the nurses and doctors for assistance. So they just wait until I ask for them.

What does it mean to feel *kreng jai*? Something like the flip side of gratitude, *kreng jai* is a common but tricky term that expresses what many people feel about receiving care from the public hospital. This everyday Thai expression, whose meaning puzzles many nonnative speakers, has been translated into English as "the feeling of embarrassment in the presence of powerful people" (Van Esterik 2000, 39), "consideration" (Kamol Somvichian 1976, 155), and "an attitude of modesty and deference that aims to avoid disturbing others" (Weisz et al. 1987, 720). To understand the subtleties of this expression, it is important to note that although *khwam kreng jai*, a sense of humbleness and politeness, can be used in a broad range of social contexts in Thailand where consideration must be given to proper manners, the social relations and knowledge that are embedded in the expression can differ greatly. Van Esterik explains using the Thai metaphor *kalatesa* that one's sense of social appropriateness is defined by one's contextual sensitivity to time, space, and knowledge about the people and situations with which one interacts.[10] Therefore, in this Thai notion of social positioning, there are no written rules and protocols for proper behavior, but instead people constantly read social cues "in such delicate juxtaposition that a slight shift in time or space alters the experience" (Van Esterik 2000, 40).

My concern is with how this specific emotion is constituted in the social fabric of the public hospital. While the hospital as a waiting place induces complex feelings related to relief, discomfort, hope, and disappointment, *kreng jai* articulates a specific relational mode of navigating this space to receive care and treatment. As with other social norms, *kreng jai* is what people instantly feel but also are socially obliged to feel at the hospital. What does this specific affect, *kreng jai*, a mixture of embarrassment, humbleness, and masking, tell us about people's experience of using health services?

During the young father's final days in Ban Phaet, Nuwan and the patient's wife once told me that they accepted the situation (*tham jai*): this acceptance related not only to the family's preparedness for the impending death but also to their lack of power to negotiate with the hospital staff, as Nuwan explained, because of *kreng jai*.[11] The family could not demand any further care from the public hospital system even though they were desperate to find a way to save the patient. So they went to a private hospital, where they would not need to feel *kreng jai* and could directly buy care and treatment services, but the cost went beyond the limits of what their ordinary rural family could afford. Hierarchical relations between the medical staff and the patient's family would be largely similar in private and public hospitals, but in a public hospital, those receiving care for themselves or family members feel constrained because they are positioned as "taking what one is given solely and having no voice in the selection or the decision" (Bauman 1998, 59). In the case of the young father's treatment, both patient and family had no choice but to accept the bureaucratically administered process of care and their prescribed positions relative to the hospital's command structure.

In public hospitals, this specific sense of occupying an inferior social position impacts people's conduct at varying moments. There is some truth to the interpretation that poor people perceive the need to adopt a reserved and constrained attitude toward hospital staff because they are disempowered, but this assumption fails to address the subtlety that people express through *kreng jai*. This practical sense of social space is also closely related to what Bourdieu called "knowledge without concepts" (1984, 470). In the hospital, people are not always directly oppressed or disciplined so as to cause them to act in a certain way, but the implicit expectation that they will feel *kreng jai* is palpable. As Bourdieu put it, "One's relationship to the social world and to one's proper place in it is never more clearly expressed than in the space and time one feels entitled to take from others" (1984, 474). When taking from others in the form of receiving care and treatment from a public hospital, one slides into the uncomfortable nexus of entitlement and debt. The desire to have and to know is counterbalanced by anxiousness over receiving. In the following, I draw on examples of how Shan migrants navigate public health care focusing on unsettling tensions around indebtedness and the unrequited gift.

The Unrequited Gift, or Bad Debt

It had been a long and difficult two months for Nun, a Shan migrant mother. She had given birth to her premature twins in an emergency room at a district hospital far away from Chiang Mai City, and just after delivery, her babies were transferred to the Ban Phaet Hospital neonatal intensive care unit. Nun felt very lucky that her babies could be offered intensive medical care, but she had been concerned about their medical bills. During her two-month stay in the NICU, she once asked me the estimated cost, but she was too *kreng jai* to ask nurses about money matters. Finally, the moment of truth came when her twins were ready to be discharged. A NICU nursed asked Nun to go to the cashier counter and to pay her bill. Nun and I went down there together.

A young cashier asked whether Nun had a health insurance card, and Nun showed the cashier her expired working permit. Then Nun put 1,000 baht on the table and explained that she did not have any more money. Looking at the receipts together with Nun, I could read that the total payment she had to make was around 150,000 baht (USD 4,800). From behind her glass screen, and in soft northern tones, the cashier consoled Nun, saying that she did not have to pay the bill at once. She explained that after Nun saved some money, she could return to the hospital and pay it later. Nun was then asked to sign the document titled "a promise of payback," which she did with her thumbprint.

Nun looked a bit relieved after the conversation at the cashier counter ended. She returned to the NICU, picked up her belongings and babies, and said good-bye to the staff. This last conversation was very brief. The nurses were busy looking after a newly admitted patient, and Nun did not have the chance to thank them. When we were waiting for a motorbike taxi at the hospital gate, I asked Nun what she thought about her unpaid hospital bill. "I really don't have money to pay the bill. It's huge. But, if I can, I want to pay some of it. Nurses in the NICU treated us very well, and now I know that being a nurse is not an easy job. They also work hard. If I have money, I'll repay," she replied.

For me, it was notable that the hospital cashier did not make any negative comments to Nun. When I returned to the cashier and asked what she thought about the mother from the NICU leaving her bill unpaid, she remarked, "It has been quite common since we've had the NICU. As you see, the cost of treatment at the NICU is really expensive. People who don't have a 30-baht card, most of them are migrants and from hill tribes. They are poor people. We cannot ask them to pay it all like private hospitals do. Government hospitals are not like private hospitals." The cashier's answer fully reflected the institution's position toward its own duty of care as discussed in chapter 1: "What could we do? Sick babies came to us, and our hospital belongs to the government. We should provide care for everyone." According to one hospital administrator, uninsured patients' treatment expenses were not reimbursed by the government and would eventually increase the hospital's budget deficit.

That day's discharge process indicated that Nun owed money to the hospital and that she had made a formal contract with the hospital for repayment. However, the contract in fact did not lay out any substantial legal obligation. Ban Phaet Hospital did not keep personal debt information longer than a year and only calculated the total sum of unpaid expenses. The most interesting aspect of this kind of hospital debt was that the hospital showed no strong inclination to collect the debt. When Nun's babies were admitted, there was no one who actually talked about the price of care in the NICU. Only on discharge day did the cashier let her know the expense and offer the generous deal of repayment without any interest. The nurses and doctors hardly mentioned the treatment cost to the patients, and when the patients were sent to the cashier before discharge, administrative staff allowed them to leave without making a payment or to make a loose arrangement for delayed payment.

Within the hospital, the unpaid expense of care is not an individualized debt but is instead subsumed as a part of the moral obligations of the hospital to the local community. Based on the Health Security Act and the national policies for health budget allocation, it could be a legitimate action to exclude noncitizens or nonbeneficiaries from the public health care system. However, when the debts of uninsured people are not expected to be paid and care is regarded as something that the hospital is obligated to give, the boundary between inclusion and exclusion starts to shift. In this local hospital, the imagined moral obligation of the state blurs the distinction between citizens and noncitizens and strengthens the inclusive aspects of public health.

What I came to know later was that it was not Nun's first debt to a hospital. A month after her twins' discharge, I visited her house in Fang district, two hundred kilometers away from Chiang Mai City. Nun lived in a wooden hut next to a small orange tree orchard. She had come to Thailand ten years previously and started to work at a big orange farm. After I had dinner with the family, I could see her husband's picture on the wall and realized why he could not come to the hospital to see his newly born children. One of his legs was amputated. Several years earlier, he had had a motorbike accident and undergone surgery in the Chiang Mai University Hospital. I remarked, "You must have spent a fortune after his accident." "Yes," Nun replied, "but not at the hospital. They asked us to pay back later, but after we came back home we couldn't return the money to the hospital. At that time, we didn't have a cell phone, so the hospital couldn't contact us. It was not like now." I wondered why she had worried about the hospital bill so much in the NICU, despite already having had the experience of receiving charity care. Nun assured me, "It will be okay, I guess. They will not report me to the police or do something to us. But, I'm *kreng jai* to them. Even if I can pay only just a part, I want to repay."

Here, the feeling of *kreng jai* had traveled far beyond the hospital walls and continued to impact the life of this migrant family. Nun knew through her previous experience that the hospital debt eventually could be waived, yet the sense of indebtedness lingered. I was quite struck that although the situation seemed to allow her to behave opportunistically and to simply forget about the debt, she had pondered her unbalanced relationship with the hospital. Here it is also important to note that Nun's reluctance to be indebted is imbued with a common karmic logic that presumes distinctive connections between debt, suffering, moral deservingness, and destiny.[12]

In this NICU, the hospital debt of many migrants has been transformed into a gift but one based on their fragile dependence on the public hospital and on the sympathy of the hospital staff. While the hospital generously offered care and treatment to noncitizen patients, the distinction between them and the rest of the political community was still palpable. At this contingent verge of exclusion and inclusion, Nun was grateful and *kreng jai* at the same time.

Interdependence, Freedom, and Living with Dignity

I would not want to create the impression that all public hospital users in Thailand are submissive and disempowered. The introduction of universal health coverage is based on the expansion of social rights that ensure equal access to health care, and there has been a growing number of lawsuits filed against hospitals reflecting the strengthened awareness of patients' rights.[13] Nor I do wish to claim that public health care in Thailand has created a "welfare dependent" population. In the short history of welfare in Thailand, the public infrastructure has not been comprehensive enough to realize its promise of a wide range of social benefits. What must be explained with regard to the practical implication of universal health coverage in Thailand, especially for the rural poor, is how it has unfolded as an obligatory circuit of care.

Two strands to the overall logic of the vernacularization of universal health care may therefore be identified. First, hospital users' popular understanding of universal health coverage reveals that giving care is a prominent manifestation of the legitimacy of power in the contemporary Thai political landscape. The intimate connection between the personal virtue of political authorities and the power of giving is a crucial feature of localizing social welfare in Thailand. The charitable state is a long-lasting foundation of religio-political authority in Thailand, yet there is more than paternalism at stake. In the midst of the globalized marketization of health care, the state's promising but obscure gift of care masks structural inequality and entails tensions around the contingency of care from the state.

Second, this specific mode of governing constitutes a particular type of subject. Patient waiting is a basic condition of receiving public health care. Frustration over the failure to deliver adequate care has been an important part of the reality of universal health coverage in Thailand. Yet the deeper but silent contention resides in "patience" itself. At the slippery slope of entitlement and dependence, *kreng jai*, an affective disposition of waiting and hesitance, reflects recipients' subordinate position within asymmetrical power relations. For the uninsured population, who do not have formal entitlements and are left to rely on the informal promise of universal access to health care, the tensions between the gift and debt become intense.

And in this circuit of care, competing impulses of desire and demur intersect. On the one hand, there is gratitude over receiving care; on the other, there is bitterness at being a "patient" subject who is required to wait. People place their faith in the good intentions of the medical staff and social protection from the state, but they also long for the freedom and economic means to choose between public and private health care. In a public hospital setting, the social bonds created when care is given and received are carefully managed, but at the same time this web of obligation signals a lack of power and autonomy.

Regarding this tension, we might recall Bourdieu's emphasis on the connection between gifts and dominance. The agony of people who cannot join the market transaction of care and have to rely on state aid is an experience similar to "the gentle, invisible form of violence, which is never recognized as such, and is not so much undergone as chosen, the violence of credit, confidence, obligation, personal loyalty, hospitality, gifts, gratitude, piety," identified by Bourdieu (1977, 192) as the main feature of the precapitalist economy. Patients' shouldering of the burden of being a recipient might be explained as a symptom of the consensual dimension of symbolic violence and intimate connections between care and repression. Yet the framework of violence cannot illuminate the moral autonomy displayed by those in a dependent situation. Although *kreng jai* reflects a constraint on one's actions, there is a sense in which this subtle hesitance and deference reflects less the suppression of one's agency than the pursuit of dignity in a dependent situation.

Indeed, the risk of being indebted did not arise solely from the fear of violent retaliation or alienation. Rather, people's desire to return what had been given was a way of living with dignity. Yi, a young father and Shan migrant, uninsured but with temporary resident status in Thailand, often slept on one side of the small hospital bed next to his three-year-old son. When he came to the ward after his work at the construction site, his shirt was covered with white plaster dust: working almost every day and coming to the hospital to check on his son and wife, he drooped with tiredness. When he told me that he had paid the hospital 13,000 baht (around USD 417), I wondered why he had done it. Clearly Yi knew, because of his previous experience with hospital debt, that he could remain indebted and there would be no direct consequences to him or his son. But still he was willing to pay back as much as he could. As a close friend of his family, I knew it had been very hard for him to save the 13,000 baht. When I asked him why he did not just ignore the bill, he told me, "I was not taught to live like that. If I had money, I should return it to them. I don't want to be indebted." Yi could not clear all his hospital debts, but he did the best he could. His silent determination, intersecting with an ethics of karmic responsibility—Yi's own commitment in this obligatory circuit of care—was steeped in his *kreng jai*.

On the edge of dependence and autonomy, freedom and obligation, Yi's everyday morality, his effort to achieve as much mutuality as possible, lays bare other dimensions of humbleness, self-respect, and living-with-dignity within interdependence. Although paying off his bill would not put him on equal footing with his benefactors, even this failed attempt at reciprocity represents an attempt to respond to his moral entanglement in relations of care. In multiple scales of caregiving, it is impossible for anyone to achieve like-for-like reciprocity (Leach 1982, 150–52); for example, it would be impossible to repay the gift of life-saving care.[14] And multiple sources of care create heterogeneous and multidirectional relations—domination, repression, legitimate authority, personal bonds, and the many other forms of sociality. In this complex network of entanglement, care is carefully elicited. These uneasy but tangible connections might be the groundwork for an "open-ended agreement in which each party commits itself to maintain the life of the other" (Graeber 2001, 162).

One of the key lessons from the Thai experience of universal health coverage is that the gift of care is not always an explicit form of domination or empowerment. Under the current system, people like Ruen and Yi are neither victims nor winners. After long and painful waiting, Ruen eventually received peritoneal dialysis treatment, life-saving care for end-stage renal failure. Yi repeatedly brought his uninsured son to the hospital, and his son received necessary treatment, although he never cleared his debt. In both instances needed care was given, yet being enmeshed in such relations was painful in both a physical and moral sense. Despite their different citizenship status and health problems, what Ruen and Yi shared was their insistence on securing a foothold in the domain of care. Their agentive submission and tenacious claim to being subjects of care, which I have called elicitation, invite us to see such affective enactments as a central dimension of the materialization of state aid and social assistance in the lives of the poor and to rethink interdependence not as a state but as a form of struggle.

3

Careful Inscription

An Ordinary Birth

On August 1, 2010, Pha, a twenty-six-year-old Shan woman, invited me to her son's first month celebration. After the bathing ritual for her baby to wish him good health and well-being, family members and guests tied a white string around his wrist with words of blessing and gifts of small banknotes.[1] Cotton threads bound the baby's young fickle soul to his body and connected the baby to his family members and neighbors.[2] I had met Pha at the antenatal clinic in a small government hospital where Pha had visited regularly during her pregnancy. Since our initial interview in the clinic, I developed a close relationship with most of Pha's extended family members in Chiang Mai. Pha's family had moved from Shan State in Myanmar to Thailand at different times during the last two decades and had various types of residency statuses. Pha's mother was an undocumented migrant; Pha's brother had a "Highlander Card," a special form of identification given to ethnic minorities who do not have Thai citizenship; Pha's husband had a "Ten-Year Card," another special form of identification for stateless people; and Pha had a working permit as a documented migrant worker. That day, I wondered: What would this one-month-old baby's own identity be? What kind of citizenship status would be given to Pha's son?

Pha's answer was clear and simple. The baby had a chance of becoming a Thai citizen not because he was born in Thailand but because he had a birth certificate from the hospital. Pha showed me a pack of documents concerning her son: an antenatal logbook, a hospital card for the baby, the baby's first picture presented to Pha by the hospital, and a birth registration certificate from the district office, all of which were neatly packed in a plastic folder. In this chapter, I explore how such a set of documents related to pregnancy and birth becomes an object of desire and hope for Shan migrants. In this mixed status migrant family, the threat of statelessness looms large with the birth of a new family member. While the various sorts of identification given to Pha's family members indicate their differentiated membership relative to the nation-state, here the baby's birth documents are presented as offering a genuine possibility for obtaining citizenship. Tracing the ways in which pregnancy records and birth-related papers are produced and imagined at the margins of the state, I attempt to unravel how the very fact of birth is constituted within the process of elicitation.

The situation of the newly born baby from a Shan migrant family is particularly pertinent for understanding the link between human life and sovereignty. Whereas one can become a subject of a sovereign state or a member of a nation by birth, "the continuity between man and citizen, nativity and nationality," what philosopher Giorgio Agamben calls the "originary fiction of modern sovereignty" (1998, 128), breaks down in the case of undocumented migrants, temporary residents, stateless people, and refugees. The uncertainty and insecurity that Pha's family went through can be assimilated to Agamben's notion of "bare life," a human life in states of exception. Rethinking sovereignty as realized over life itself, he distinguishes a political being, endowed with a form of life proper to an individual or a group, from bare life, life stripped of its political and social qualities. In his book *Homo Sacer* (1998), he suggests that modern sovereign power is demonstrated through ways of both including and excluding bare life from its polity. Rather than assuming the new baby's life as being inherently deprived of any political attribute, I focus on the political stakes of giving birth to a noncitizen and on the gestures made in recognition of this birth. The main question I address is not how one can be violently stripped of political being at the start of a life but how one who starts from the realm of the exception elicits care and slips into the domain of the political.

On their auspicious celebration day, Pha's family showed me two ways of binding. The white cotton thread for the first-month initiation ritual signifies the baby's inclusion in the basic social relations of kinship and local community. This ritual brings a newly born baby into the domestic and social world of nurturance. The other binding takes place between personal and documentary forms of life: everyday human existence is also attached to a paper life in the sphere of bureaucratic state administration.[3] This binding of the personal to the bureaucratic matters particularly to ambiguous political subjects, whose belonging to nation-states is partial and uncertain.[4]

Among the numerous places that produce bureaucratic documentation, the antenatal clinic offers an interesting venue to observe how paper-mediated binding starts from the very beginning of human life. By focusing on the routine procedure of antenatal care and its aftereffects, I trace the ways in which the fact of birth is constituted and valued in the context of transnational migration and displacement. Critical attention has been paid to birth as a site of political contestations over the bearing and raising of a new generation, including close explorations of how biomedical technologies, state policies, and gender relations shape reproductive meanings and practices.[5] While I focus on Shan women's reproductive struggles in this chapter, my main inquiry is not into how migrant women's bodies and fertility are controlled and rendered as governable objects. Instead, I show how these women appropriate biopolitical technologies of verification and by doing so invoke a tangible relationship with the state. I suggest that reflecting on people's concerted efforts to overcome "the status of an uncountable excluded subject" (Honneth et al. 2016, 123) allows a new perspective on reproduction and care as a groundwork for the emergence of a political subject.

I begin by examining the convoluted documentation processes imposed on migrants in Thailand to understand the efficacy of unofficial identification papers. Then I turn to Ban Phaet Hospital and demonstrate the predominance of Shan women in the clinic by analyzing the patterns of their antenatal attendance. The necessary partnership between Shan mothers and nurses to complete this particular course of care shows that legibility is not imposed but acquired through shared labor. Birth certificates for migrant children, in this context, serve as a lens through which to analyze noncitizen subjects' assertion of their political relationship with the state.

The Uncountable: Shan Migrants in Chiang Mai

The strong presence of Shan communities in northern Thailand is not a new phenomenon. However, economic malaise and political suppression in Myanmar and labor shortages in the low-skilled sector in Thailand since the 1980s have led to a mass migration of Shan people. The difficult living and working conditions experienced by Shan and other migrants from Myanmar in Thailand have been addressed with a special focus on labor exploitation; exclusion from health care and social welfare services; and harassment and abuse from employers, the police, and border patrols.[6]

Within the landscape of Chiang Mai, it is problematic to consider migrant status as something neatly defined by legal terms and procedures that undergird a self-evident set of entitlements. As the complex migration history of Pha's family members reveals, administrative and legal ambiguity characterizes the contemporary regime of authorized migration. The state's attempts to sort out noncitizen subjects in the sovereign territory have resulted in a proliferation of varying types of identity documents. Yet, as anthropological discussions about documented lives suggest, the state's writing practices not only make people more legible and governable; they also create spaces of uncertainty and indeterminacy in which people negotiate the gaps between their physical and documented selves.[7]

As migrant policies evolve in Thailand, two aspects are crucial to the social and legal constitution of non-Thai others, including ethnic minorities and migrants. First, there have been many different types of noncitizens, and this has blurred the lines between refugees and migrants, political and economic factors, and forced and voluntary migration. Since 1965, eighteen or more identification cards with different titles, colors, issuing places, authorizing bodies, and expiration conditions have been issued to non-Thai nationals and people who have difficulty in establishing their nationality (the "stateless") in Thailand (Pinkaew Laungaramsri 2014). Since then, various special types of ID cards have become legal vehicles that facilitate the long-term stay of numerous people who cross the border without proper documents (Keyes 2002; Toyota 2005).

Second, the poorly planned and inconsistent documentation process plays a significant role in producing undocumented migrants. Since 1992, the Thai government has allowed temporary residency for those migrants who entered Thai soil "illegally" and has issued work permits for a two-year period (Migrant Assistance Programme Foundation 2012). Although migrant workers were registered and documented through this yearly amnesty program, in the eyes of the law, they still lack legal status because of the illegal way in which they gained entry (Hall 2011). At the end of each two-year period, deportations as well as the renewal of working permits occurred regularly. In 2007 a system for verifying nationality and creating temporary passports was initiated, and many Shan migrants expected that

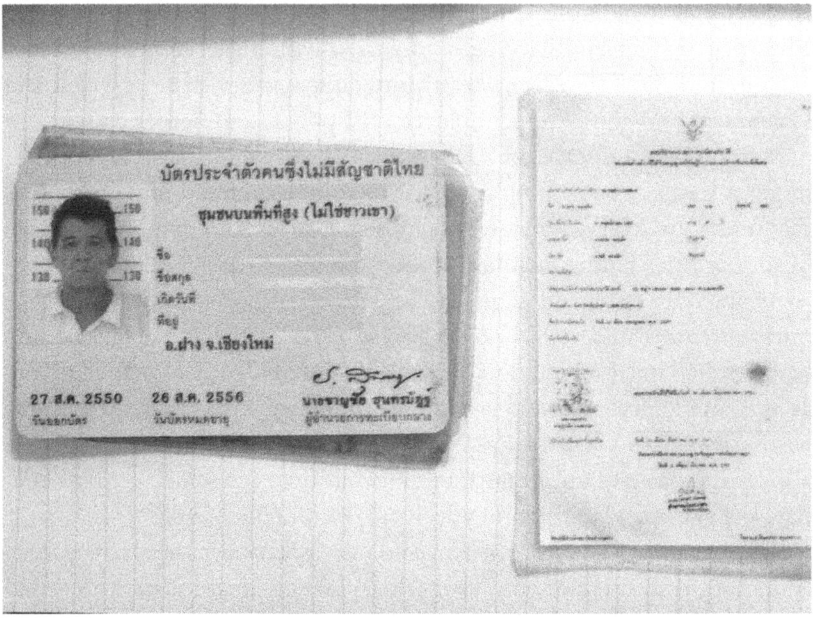

Figure 3. Different forms of identification for non-Thai citizens

these passports would ensure their ability to remain in Thailand long-term and travel freely throughout the country.

By September 2013, around 1.7 million migrants from Myanmar had gained temporary passports following the new rules (Nyein Nyein 2013a); however, these temporary passports warranted only four-year working visas. By the end of 2013, about 400,000 of the total number of registered migrants from Myanmar were already facing the end of their working visas (Nyein Nyein 2013b; O'Toole 2013a, 2013b). The Thai government agreed to extend the permission given to labor migrants to stay for another two years in 2013, yet it did not propose any long-term plan for these temporary passport holders. Since 2015, the six-year working visa has begun to expire, and some formally documented migrants are now on the verge of becoming illegal and undocumented aliens (Migrant Workers Rights Network 2015).[8]

These legislative changes have caused many Shan people in Thailand to oscillate between documented and undocumented status. Here it is important to note that not only formal working permits and passports but also any sorts of identifying documents can have the effect of making an individual legible in the eyes of the state. For migrants, the state can be an object of both fear and attachment (Aretxaga 2003; Das and Poole 2004), and this subjective dynamic of intimacy and distance is well reflected in the Shan migrants' desire to have identification documents. Shan people not only strategically avoid encounters with state agents who can abruptly exercise their powers to arrest, detain, and deport them; they also try to keep certain connections with state agents through quasi-official documents that make them recognizable.

To think through this specific attachment between migrants and the state, migrant women's experience of giving birth to and raising a child opens up a new field of inquiry. Within the current legal framework, which regards the adult migrant worker as the only legitimate subject of authorized migration, Thailand does not have any formal identification systems for migrant children. In this context, rather than letting their children remain in the shadows, Shan parents actively gather papers related to the evidence of birth that can make their children legible. Some of them hope that their children might have a chance to become Thai citizens through proof of their birth in Thailand.[9] Others do not share this dream but still want to have whatever documents they can obtain concerning their children. In the following, I delve into Shan women's access to antenatal care and discuss how they adopt this biomedical practice as a possible way of procuring documents.

Antenatal Care for All

Maternal and child health is one of the most prominent areas that demonstrate the effectiveness of the Thai public health care system. Due to the nationwide introduction of primary health care and improved family planning, the infant mortality rate decreased from 46 per 1,000 live births in 1980 to 7.7 in 2005 (McGuire 2010, 311). Also, the coverage of antenatal and delivery care by a skilled health worker increased to around 97 percent by 2006 (Supon Limwattananon et al. 2010). In terms of the migrant population, from 2004 to 2006, around 33,300 new births were reported to the Ministry of Public Health, and more than 90 percent of them were delivered by health personnel within public health facilities (Samrit Srithamrongsawat et al. 2010).[10]

The antenatal clinic of Ban Phaet Hospital provides a comprehensive picture of Shan women's utilization of maternal health care services from the public health care system. The most noteworthy feature of maternal health care in this hospital is the predominance of Shan migrant women in situ. From 2007 to 2010, 1,395 women visited Ban Phaet Hospital antenatal clinic, and around 45 percent of them were Shan migrants, including both those who were documented and those who were not (see table 1).[11] Documented migrants who were covered by the compulsory migrant health insurance were eligible to access antenatal and delivery care by paying 30 baht for each visit, but migrants who were not covered by the CMHI and those who do not have a Thai national ID card were required to pay out-of-pocket expenses.[12] Nurses in their everyday practices did not distinguish between documented and undocumented migrants in terms of services provided, and the basic procedure for antenatal care was the same regardless of one's insurance status.

The basic pattern of antenatal attendance observed in Ban Phaet Hospital's antenatal clinic demonstrates that Shan women access more antenatal services than Thai women. Compared to Thai women who are covered by the universal health coverage, the proportion of migrant women who visited the clinic in the first trimester of pregnancy is slightly smaller; nevertheless,

Table 1. Total visits to Ban Phaet Hospital antenatal care from October 2007 to September 2010

	Oct. 2007–Sep. 2008		*Oct. 2009–Sep. 2010*		*Oct. 2009–Sep. 2010*	
Health insurance status	*Total number*	*%*	*Total number*	*%*	*Total number*	*%*
Civil servant health insurance plan	3	0.8	5	1	2	0.4
UC—registered to Ban Phaet Hospital	120	31	173	33	157	32
UC—not registered to Ban Phaet Hospital	62	16.2	57	11	47	9.6
Migrant—including both documented and undocumented migrants	174	45	246	47	220	45
Social security plan for formal sector workers	24	6	43	8	62	13
Total	383		524		488	

the Shan women subsequently attended the antenatal clinic more often. Of the total number of women who attended the clinic more than four times, Shan were more numerous than any other group of women.[13] Another noticeable fact is that civil servant health insurance beneficiaries, a segment of the middle class, rarely used the public hospital, despite being able to access antenatal care free of charge. This pattern coincides with Thai middle-class women's general preference for private facilities over public hospitals.

In fact, the migrant women in my study had the highest rate of attendance, with nearly a quarter of them making more than ten visits (see table 2). This pattern is explained by the fact that Shan women tended to keep most of their monthly and weekly scheduled checkups, while several Thai women often missed their appointments. The other noticeable difference is that the proportion of migrant women who started to visit the antenatal clinic in the later stage of pregnancy—after twenty-one weeks of pregnancy—is much smaller than the corresponding proportion of Thai women (see table 3). In the overall pattern of antenatal visits, women in the migrant category used the public service more actively and properly according to the national guidelines for antenatal care.

Long Journey to the Clinic: Compliance and Accountability

Faithful compliance with the antenatal care process as shown by the Shan migrant mothers is deeply related to their aspirations to have a better life in Thailand. For many Shan women who originally came from rural areas in Myanmar, the antenatal clinic often became the first place where they

Table 2. Number of antenatal care visits in Ban Phaet Hospital from October 2007 to September 2010

		Numbers of antenatal care visits							
		1		*2–3*		*4–9*		*>9*	
Insurance status	*Total number*	*Number of people*	*%*	*Number of people*	*%*	*Number of people*	*%*	*Number of people*	*%*
UC—registered to Ban Phaet Hospital	450	66	14.67	102	22.67	215	47.78	67	14.89
Migrant	640	64	10	93	14.53	330	51.56	153	23.91

Table 3. Timing of first antenatal visit, Ban Phaet Hospital Antenatal Clinic, October 2007 to September 2010

		Numbers of antenatal care visits							
		0–12		*13–20*		*21–31*		*32+*	
Insurance status	*Total number*	*Number of people*	*%*	*Number of people*	*%*	*Number of people*	*%*	*Number of people*	*%*
UC—registered to Ban Phaet Hospital	450	154	34.22	145	32.22	113	25.11	38	8.44
Migrant	640	218	34.06	276	43.13	117	18.28	29	4.53

experienced modern and well-established medical procedures. Sen, a thirty-year-old Shan woman, gave birth after ten visits to Ban Phaet Hospital's antenatal clinic. As Sen explained why she had not missed any appointments, she went on to relate her past birth experience. Sen had given birth to her first baby deep in the jungle, while accompanying her husband, who was involved in the Shan State Army. She had had to give birth on her own, without any assistance, and her son had died shortly after being born. Sen told me once: "If I could have given birth in a hospital like this in Thailand, my baby would not have died. . . . I wanted to do everything right this time. Here, nurses take care of pregnant women well. They are interested in whether my baby grows up properly, set appointments for checkups, and they give me medicine too." While most Shan women I met perceived hospital birth as a desirable and normative practice, some of them emphasized that antenatal care was a prerequisite for accessing hospital birth in Thailand. They were told that if they did not go to hospital for antenatal checkups but only for delivery, nurses would criticize them and possibly refuse to provide them with a delivery certificate. Although many women complained about long waiting times, antenatal and maternal care was frequently mentioned as the most beneficial service that they had ever received from Thai public hospitals. As I continued to meet Shan women who were pregnant or had given birth in Thailand, what I came to understand was that the benefit of accessing antenatal care often went further than simply receiving modern biomedical care. During their pregnancies, migrant women were constantly asked to return to the clinic, and such an invitation itself was highly appreciated as it signaled the medical staff's attention and concern for their welfare.

Maew was among the many Shan women who had diligently kept their appointments. A nineteen-year-old Shan woman, she gave birth for the first time after nine visits to Ban Phaet Hospital's antenatal clinic. She had moved to Thailand with her sister-in-law when she was twelve years old and had never had the chance to go to school. Like many Shan women, Maew never missed an appointment, yet her dedication was especially striking: for each visit, she spent almost four hours traveling to the clinic by public transport. In the last month of her pregnancy, she visited the hospital every week. To make these trips, she left her house at 6 a.m. to avoid the busy waiting lines at the hospital and then returned to her house under the sweltering midday sun, changing minibuses three times.

Maew's determination to attend the antenatal clinic lay somewhere in between what she desired and what she felt obligated to do. Looking at her antenatal logbook, in which all the tables were perfectly completed, I asked why she had not missed a single appointment. She laughed at my question and then tried to explain something she saw as obvious.

> The nurse would definitely scold me if I hadn't come to the clinic. Also, if I hadn't come to the clinic each time the nurse asked, my baby would not grow properly [*mai sombun*]. If you want to have a healthy baby and want to give birth without any problems, you have to come to the hospital all the time. And if I hadn't kept my appointments, the nurses would not have taken responsibility and given us documents. It's very important.

In Maew's account, participation in the routines of antenatal care was something that generated trust. The nurses' request was not only understood as a rule that she had to follow but also the basis of shared accountability with the nurses. As Maew noted, the hierarchy between the nurses and mothers is not something that can be easily dismissed, yet her compliance and that of other Shan women does not simply indicate their passivity under imposed rules. Rather, they are working on a way to secure care and to receive public validation of the birth of their babies.

Mutual Obligation to Care

The contradiction embodied by Ban Phaet Hospital's antenatal clinic is that this government facility, whose purpose is to provide health care to Thai citizens, in fact mostly serves non-Thai others. When I asked Nurse Pu, an experienced obstetric nurse in her forties, to comment on the high proportion of Shan migrants at the clinic, she replied instantly, "No problem. They are adorable."

It was late afternoon, just before the clinic's closing time. It had been a busy day for her. That day, twenty-six women had visited the antenatal clinic, and Nurse Pu had also arranged a referral to the provincial hospital for a teenage mother who had developed symptoms of premature birth. In this clinic, only three nurses and two nurses' aides handled the provision of antenatal care, vaccinations for children, and managing the labor room. Women who came to the hospital at around 8 a.m. would wait for between one and two hours in the waiting chairs before being seen. When demand was high, the nurses had to ask women who arrived late in the morning to come back after lunch. Most of those who came early in the morning were Shan women. Nurse Pu explained:

> Most Shan women, they are really good mothers. They listen to us, and are willing to know how to take care of their pregnancy. They keep their appointment dates without fail. When we advise them about good eating habits during pregnancy and breastfeeding, they really try to follow what we teach them. . . . Sometimes, Thai women are too stubborn, and they are not really interested in what we are saying. It's quite understandable, because they are surrounded by their parents, aunts, and grandmothers who tell them what they should eat and all other kinds of things. But these Shan women are not like that. They have moved far away from home, live in a nuclear family in Thailand, and there is no one who can help them if something happens. These people are relying on us, and it's very rewarding to provide antenatal care to Shan women.

Nurse Pu's comparison between Thai and Shan mothers reflects a changing local landscape in which Shan migrant women have become a major party calling for the transaction of care. As Nurse Pu confirmed the clinic's openness to Shan women, it is important to note that in her explanation, the typical attributes of migrants—lack of education and social support, and economic hardship—were converted to a readiness to accept new knowledge and rules. Keeping appointment dates, bringing their antenatal logbooks with them, and paying attention to nurses' advice were voluntary efforts made by the Shan women that the nurses valued highly and interpreted as good qualities for a mother to have.

The nurses are well aware of the illegality embedded in migrant status and the vulnerable position of Shan women, yet in this clinic no logic of exclusion negates the state's obligation to care. While the comparison between Thai and Shan women thus emphasizes the otherness attached to Shan migrants, here it hardly undermines the deservingness of migrant women as legitimate subjects of care. As Nurse Pu asserted, "We have to take care of everyone equally whether they are insured or not. If babies could not be born safely, the government should be responsible." Throughout the daily practices of the nurses, it is not a matter of whether migrant women have the right to access health care. It is, rather, that ensuring a safe birth is the obligation of the state, and that the nurses are active conveyors of this idealized mode of governing. Here, the nurses' daily practices enact an inclusive relationship between the state and noncitizen others.

One important aspect of antenatal care is its role in generating biomedical information about noncitizens that can then be used for the bureaucratic purpose of monitoring. A key aim of antenatal care is to monitor and intervene in woman's bodies to ensure a healthy pregnancy. During this procedure, antenatal checkups operate as a means of producing a record regarding the parents and fetus. Information gathered in the logbook includes details of biological traits and changes that take place in the pregnant woman's body (weight, blood pressure, urinary glucose, and protein levels); thalassemia screening is offered; and previous miscarriages and abortion experiences are also recorded.

Above all else, the names of the mother and father are identified and documented through antenatal care. While enrolling one's name in a register is a basic procedure for any bureaucratic and medical work, this routine verification indeed plays a crucial role in documenting the fact of birth. To do this, the nurses take extra precautions in checking the migrant mother's ID and preventing claims of fake paternity. Whenever a Shan mother lacks any kind of documentation, the nurses request a mugshot and keep the picture for further identification purposes. The nurses also refuse to record the father's name in the antenatal logbook and subsequently in the delivery certificate unless the pregnant woman—whether Thai or Shan—has brought the baby's biological father to the clinic or provided the father's ID card. A nurse who mainly organized pre–blood test counseling for expecting parents explained: "We need to record everything correctly. Otherwise the baby's birth document will contain misleading information."

In this particular form of reproductive regime, it is important to note that the nurses' scrutinizing gaze is not something all-encompassing and predominating. To do their jobs properly, nurses are inherently dependent on the mothers' cooperation because they cannot coerce the mothers into attending each and every antenatal session and complying with all bureaucratic procedures. Here, the medicalization of pregnancy requires allegiances between the mother and the state agent. The partnership between the nurses and Shan mothers reveals that in this specific context, "seeing like a state," a project of verification and legibility (Scott 1998), is a shared task: the nurses try to produce correct and accurate information for each birth, and Shan mothers attempt to make their children's births both safe and visible. Within this mutual dependence, Shan migrant mothers' faithful involvement not only demonstrates a certain process of subjectivization by the biomedical authority but also speaks to their own capacity to be a part of the medical and bureaucratic system of counting.[14] In this context, antenatal care exercises a form of governmentality that is constituted through mutual obligation rather than through a panoptic gaze of surveillance.

The Birth Certificate and Its Double Reading

The long and hectic journeys to the antenatal clinic are carefully recorded in an antenatal logbook, and it is this specific record that eventually holds the power of recognition and identification. The last page of the antenatal logbook is the delivery certificate form, and this chronological arrangement of the medical records makes several Shan women think that antenatal care is a precondition for birth registration. Among several documents that are requested for birth registration, such as a copy of the parent's ID card and house registration and a copy of the employee's ID card and house registration, the delivery certificate from the hospital is the most essential requirement. In the female ward of the Ban Phaet Hospital, nurses advise new mothers' husbands or family members to register the baby's birth at the district office while the mothers remain in the ward as part of their recovery. Most migrant parents also regard birth registration as a serious matter and follow the advice offered by the medical staff. After childbirth, this logbook is continuously requested during home visits occasionally organized by nurses for postpartum care and at vaccination clinics.

Efforts made by Shan mothers to keep a logbook and other birth documents are based on their acute understanding of the authoritative effects of antenatal care that can result in their child's birth being recognized by the

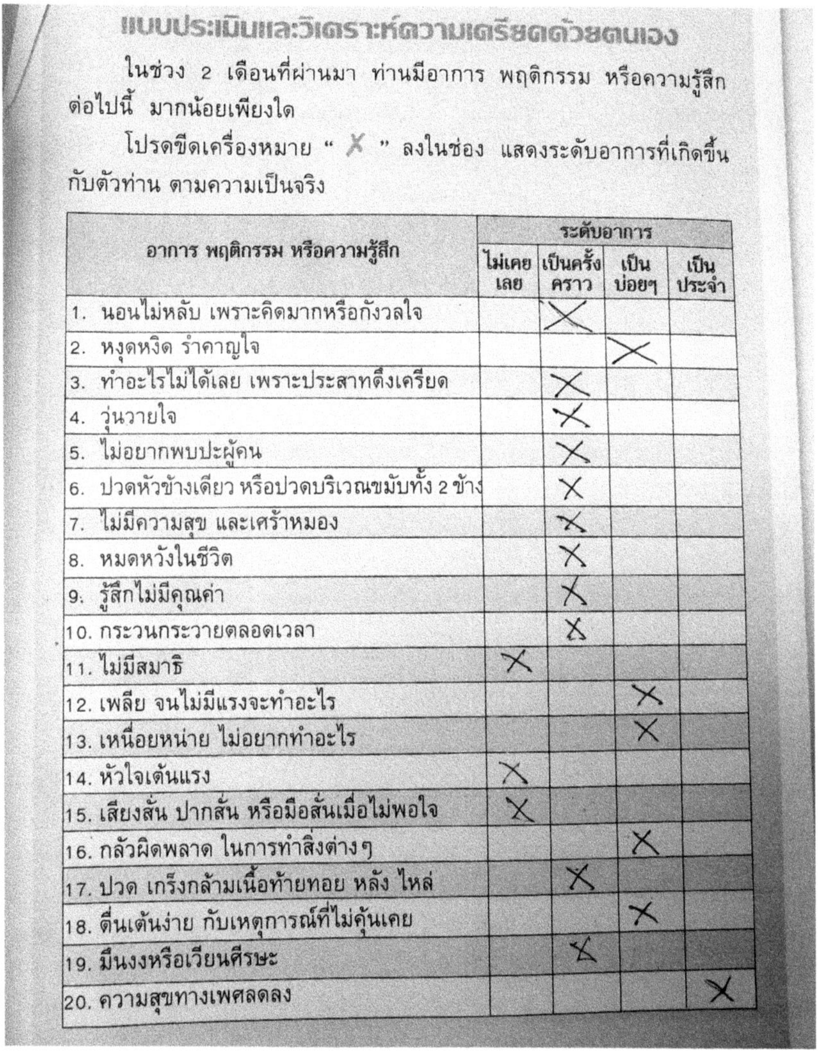

แบบประเมินและวิเคราะห์ความเครียดด้วยตนเอง

ในช่วง 2 เดือนที่ผ่านมา ท่านมีอาการ พฤติกรรม หรือความรู้สึก ต่อไปนี้ มากน้อยเพียงใด

โปรดขีดเครื่องหมาย " X " ลงในช่อง แสดงระดับอาการที่เกิดขึ้นกับตัวท่าน ตามความเป็นจริง

อาการ พฤติกรรม หรือความรู้สึก	ระดับอาการ			
	ไม่เคยเลย	เป็นครั้งคราว	เป็นบ่อยๆ	เป็นประจำ
1. นอนไม่หลับ เพราะคิดมากหรือกังวลใจ		X		
2. หงุดหงิด รำคาญใจ			X	
3. ทำอะไรไม่ได้เลย เพราะประสาทตึงเครียด		X		
4. วุ่นวายใจ		X		
5. ไม่อยากพบปะผู้คน		X		
6. ปวดหัวข้างเดียว หรือปวดบริเวณขมับทั้ง 2 ข้าง		X		
7. ไม่มีความสุข และเศร้าหมอง		X		
8. หมดหวังในชีวิต		X		
9. รู้สึกไม่มีคุณค่า		X		
10. กระวนกระวายตลอดเวลา		X		
11. ไม่มีสมาธิ	X			
12. เพลีย จนไม่มีแรงจะทำอะไร			X	
13. เหนื่อยหน่าย ไม่อยากทำอะไร			X	
14. หัวใจเต้นแรง	X			
15. เสียงสั่น ปากสั่น หรือมือสั่นเมื่อไม่พอใจ	X			
16. กลัวผิดพลาด ในการทำสิ่งต่างๆ			X	
17. ปวด เกร็งกล้ามเนื้อท้ายทอย หลัง ไหล่		X		
18. ตื่นเต้นง่าย กับเหตุการณ์ที่ไม่คุ้นเคย			X	
19. มึนงงหรือเวียนศีรษะ		X		
20. ความสุขทางเพศลดลง				X

Figure 4. A self-diagnosis table for postpartum depression. Migrant women who cannot read Thai reported that they checked this table with help from their children or friends who know Thai. During my observations in the antenatal clinic, nurses never directly asked their clients to fill out this form, but some of my interlocutors were keen to do so. The Shan woman who answered this form checked that she "often" (third column) became edgy (no. 2), had little energy to do to anything due to exhaustion (no. 12), felt lethargic (no. 13), and found herself easily upset in unfamiliar situations (no. 18).

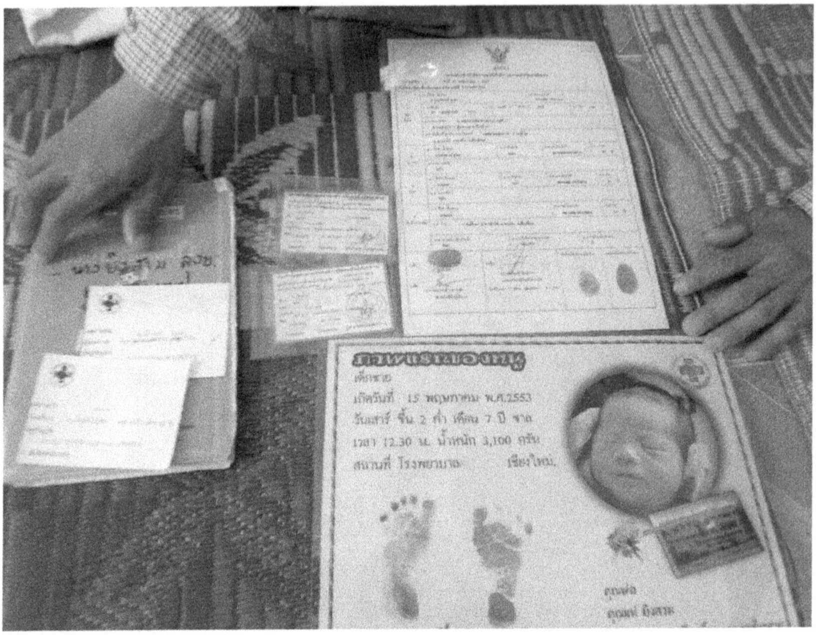

Figure 5. A Shan mother's documents related to her baby's birth (*clockwise from left*): an antenatal logbook, the parents' Migrant Worker Cards, a birth registration document from the district office, and the baby's picture from the hospital.

Thai bureaucratic system. Even though many Shan women cannot read and do not know what exactly is written in their antenatal logbooks and other documents they receive from the hospital—such as hospital cards, receipts, and referral letters—they fully recognize how these documents can be used as a certain social currency inside the system. Even when a Shan mother cannot write or read her child's name in Thai, she has a written record for her child and therefore a means of navigating the busy hospital, immigration, and district offices. Many Shan women agree that the value of keeping the antenatal logbook and birth certificate is high, especially for school enrollment, and they make an effort not only to maintain the book but also to keep it safe.[15] In Shan women's houses, often at construction sites, it is easy to see these logbooks and other important documents stored in thick plastic bags, hanging under the shabby crossbeams to prevent them from being soaked by water or misplaced.

Shan parents who have a temporary resident status give particular weight to the proper birth registration in the expectation that their children may receive Thai citizenship in the future. Sing, a Shan woman in her midthirties, had a "Highlanders Card" and was very proud that she had properly managed her first son's birth registration and the subsequent household registration process with the help of the village headman.[16] She explained to me:

> When he reaches fifteen years, he can apply for a Thai identification card, because we already have his birth registration and have prepared all the documents required of him. This is the most valuable thing that we can give him as parents. When we are all gone, he will have his Thai nationality, and can have his own car and house in his name. We could never have these things, but his future will be different from what we experienced.

In contrast to Sing, Tui, another Shan woman, regretted the mistake she had made regarding birth registration. In her makeshift house built at a construction site, she told me:

> When I was pregnant, I didn't know what I should do. It was when I had just come to Thailand. I didn't go to the antenatal clinic and just went to the hospital to give birth. At that time, I didn't have much money to pay the hospital bill, so the nurse told me to come back later with money and get my delivery certificate. But I didn't go back. I wish I had paid the money even now to get my son's birth certificate back.

She then showed me the hospital wristband given to her first son at the time of his birth, on which her son's name and patient number were handwritten. She had kept this for almost eight years just in case. Tui knew that, considering her undocumented status, the birth registration would not enable her son to receive Thai citizenship. Yet what she bemoaned was her missed opportunity to give her son documentation. Having experienced the yearly renewal of working permits and frequent police inspections, she was now much more aware of the sense of security that birth documents could give her son.

As the set of documentation required for birth registration demonstrates a specific link between the newly born baby and national collectivity, it is important to note that the legal implication of birth certificates for noncitizens is still obscure. The basic difference in birth registration forms of Thai and non-Thai citizens is that if parents are not Thai nationals, then there is no section to indicate their child's nationality. This is because all Thailand-born children, regardless of their parents' legal status, can be registered in the national civil registration system according to the Civil Registration Act (2008), but this procedure does not confer any nationality (Johnson et al. 2015, 115). A subsequent problem is that if Shan children who were born in Thailand then move to Myanmar, they may not be eligible for Myanmar citizenship.[17] Within this legal indeterminacy, the birth registration in Thailand is an imperfect measure to protect Shan children from the ultimate threat of statelessness.

What I want to emphasize here is the basic ambiguity between statelessness and citizenship embedded in the birth certificates for children of noncitizens. On the one hand, birth registration legally establishes the existence of newly born Shan babies, signaling the principle that they have "the right to acquire a nationality."[18] On the other hand, the birth certificate clearly indicates that these newly born babies have no nationality at the time of registration. In this context, the birth certificate for a "stateless" child is heteroglossial in the sense that it inscribes "different voices in [a] seemingly monotonous form" (Star 1999, 385). This record carries conflicting political intentions, rationalities, and enactments.

What emerges from the birth certificate as an identification document, then, is similar to what Lawrence Cohen would call an "as if relation to the contractual narrative of modern statecraft" (Cohen 2004, 167). By possessing and presenting this document, Shan migrants expect their children to be able to locate themselves within the operation of law and bureaucratic rationality, as if they were the proper subjects of the sovereign state. Here, what is significant is that when migrant mothers complete the institutionalized medical procedures of childbirth and documentation, the effect of writing technologies is not simply alienating. Many women embrace the potential benefit of documentation and, through their own engagement with biomedical and bureaucratic processes, attempt to harness the power of this paperwork. Entry into the political realm as a legible subject is an aspiration made manifest by appropriating bureaucratic technologies for one's own ends.

Inscribing and Anchoring

Tracking down the modern construction of ethnic classification in Thailand, Keyes remarks on an intriguing assumption related to the notion of Thailand as a nation (*chat Thai*): "The term *chāt* is derived from the Sanskirt/Pali term *jāti*, 'that which is given at birth'" (Keyes 2002, 1179). Only in the late nineteenth century did the word come to mean "a people who share a common heritage from the past" (Keyes 2002, 1179). The premodern meaning connecting birth and nationality resonates today with the issues facing the children of noncitizens in Thailand: What does it mean to be a citizen or a member of the nation-state by birth? What exactly is the status at birth for people at the margins of the state?

The first page of a teenage migrant mother's antenatal logbook (see figure 6), which I accidentally encountered in Ban Phaet Hospital, captures how careful inscription plays a crucial role in creating associations around liminal subjects. According to the logbook, the mother was a seventeen-year-old Shan woman. In the book entry for her, the blank where her identification number belonged indicated that she was an undocumented migrant. She had attended antenatal care six times and had given birth to a boy weighing around 2.5 kilograms. The baby boy experienced severe hypoxia and was therefore sent to the neonatal intensive care unit, while the mother stayed in the maternal ward. After the young mother was discharged, the NICU nurse contacted her several times, but the mother never returned to the hospital to see her baby. The doctor in the NICU, who showed me the logbook, was very impressed by the mother's effort to fill out this special table. The table, which had been completed by the mother, detailed each time she had felt the fetus kick during a two-month period. Usually the antenatal nurses asked a mother to complete this kind of table when abnormal symptoms were reported in the late stage of pregnancy. The mother never came to the NICU, but the intensive care for the baby was continued.

In reading this table, I realized that inscribing a record of life can be seen as something very tangible. There are numerous ways to record the condition of the fetus in this era of new reproductive technology, yet what we have here is a very simple way of doing so. The mother's engagement in recording her baby's movements may not be a particularly robust link to the juridico-political order that defines who and what the citizen is. Yet the diligent record anticipates a subject whose existence was registered already before birth. This type of record keeping is designed to monitor one's pregnancy from a distance, yet it signifies something more than its intended purpose. Here, inscription is not just a means of forcing legibility upon unruly subjects but also an act of preserving and proving one's very existence. The young mother had faithfully participated in "the enactment of

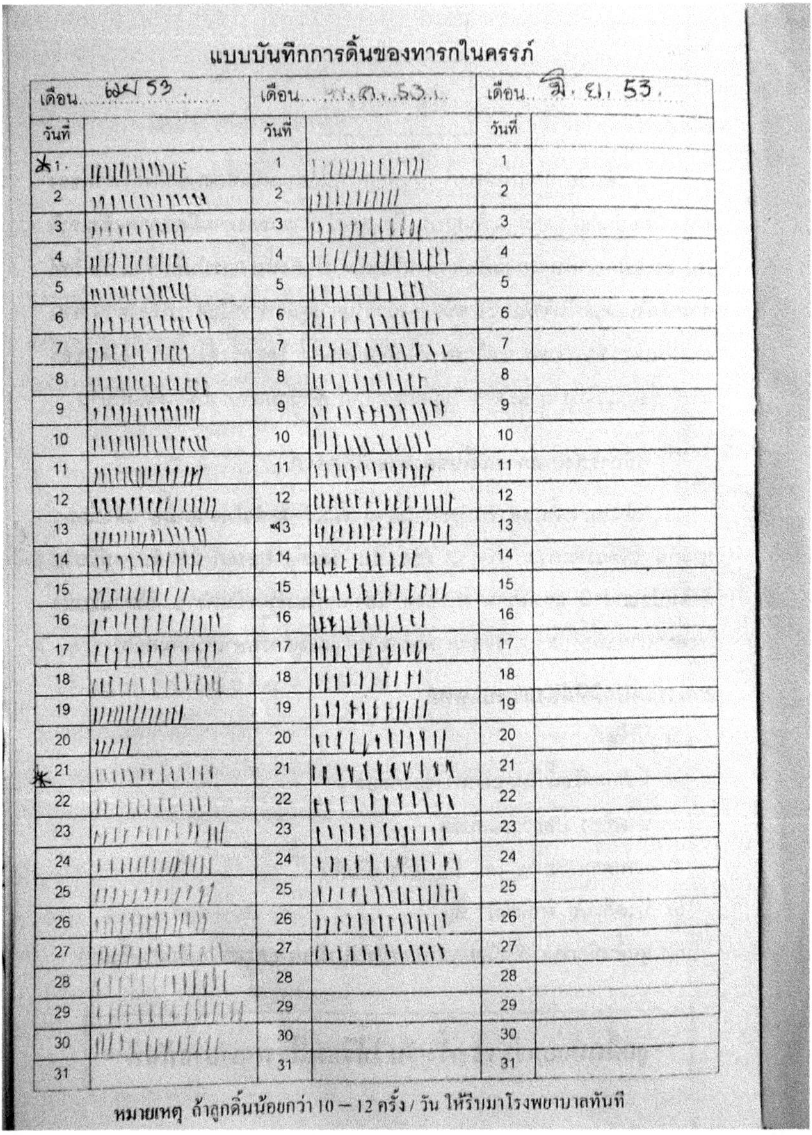

Figure 6. An antenatal care logbook in which a mother recorded fetal movement from April 2010 to May 2010

bureaucratic objects" (Hull 2012b, 18), and, as a result, this written form allowed a baby with no name and nationality to become identifiable within the wider bureaucratic associations in this space and time.

The difference between human and citizen, Jacques Rancière notes, opens "an interval for political subjectivization" and shows the "contingency of being born here or there" (Rancière 2011, 5). In this chapter, I have suggested that Shan migrant women's active participation in antenatal care shows that they acutely sense the aftereffects of this violent contingency and try to appropriate this interval through producing and accumulating associations with the hospital, bureaucratic system, and state. The work of inscription indeed has the potential to "put together a relation of inclusion and a relation of exclusion" (Rancière 2004, 304). As a medical and political process, the routines of antenatal care not only produce a certain bureaucratic truth but also ascribe identity and value to this new beginning. And accessing this mode of inscription is not restricted to the enclosed circle of medical professionals, administrators, and state bureaucrats. Illiterate migrant women become a significant part of this authorized production of information and data by accumulating, photocopying, preserving, and carrying around such state artifacts.

The documented presence that trails migrant mothers and their unborn and newly born babies thus proves how these noncitizen subjects secure partial but necessary security by creating concrete allegiances with the state. As several anthropological explorations of migrant reproduction and health suggest, the politics of illegality and deportability have perpetuated injustice and negated migrants' basic rights.[19] Being too afraid to access the hospital or to simply walk around the streets without papers characterizes many lives of migrants in Thailand and around the world in general. However, while acknowledging the analytical strength of these discussions about the embodiment of fear, anxiety, and undeservingness, I have illuminated that some everyday forms of determination cannot be discerned within the framework of abandonment and exclusion.

The very aim of inscription is indeed to preserve information so that it can be delivered later on. Although these attempts at inscription are likely to fail to negate the state's threats of disregard and expulsion, migrant women's work of inscription indicates that they and their children, numerous noncitizen subjects, are already anchored in the realm of the state bureaucracy, attempting to bridge the interstice between human and citizen.

4

Premature Life and Death

The patient in bed number 1 had been admitted a week ago, but his name was still unknown. The head nurse told me that the patient's mother was a seventeen-year-old undocumented Shan woman. The baby had experienced severe hypoxia during birth and had been sent to Ban Phaet Hospital's neonatal intensive care unit. The young mother had been advised to visit the NICU after her discharge, but she had not come to see her baby, nor had she answered nurses' repeated phone calls. This baby's most pressing problem was his fluid-filled lungs, incapable of transporting oxygen. To allow him to breathe properly, the baby was connected by several tubes and lines to a mechanical ventilator, cardiac monitor, and IV pumps; except for his regular chest movements, he lay motionless amid the tubing delivering medications, the electronic signals, and the sharp metallic beeping sounds. When the nurse pricked the sole of his foot with a needle to collect a blood sample, he did not even flinch, although the cardiac monitor beeped erratically. "*Luk, pen yangngai?*" (Son, how are you doing?), the nurse murmured as she calmed the baby by gently stroking his back. He was pricked several times a day to regularly monitor his capillary blood gas levels and set the level of ventilator support accordingly. As he lay quietly on the radiant warmer, his blood samples and X-rays made their way through the laboratory, the radiology department, and the NICU. Abundant information about him, including vital and neurological signs, medication lists, and the cost of his daily treatment were carefully recorded, sorted, and securely stored. The baby had no family around him, but his body and life were already enmeshed within complex social and ethical relations.

In this chapter, I ask about the ethical and technological modalities of care that make life and death possible in this modest NICU at Ban Phaet Hospital. As this newborn patient's parents were not present, the NICU became the single site responsible for his recovery and growth. The baby boy was uninsured, as was his migrant mother, but he was promptly resuscitated at a life-and-death moment and given scrupulous medical attention through the Thai public hospital network. By tracing the entanglement of neonate patients with medical staff, I delve into how such exceptionally vulnerable and foreign infants elicit relations of care.

As advances in neonatal technology have radically lowered the mortality of preterm and critically ill infants, neonatal care has had to deal with the problems associated with maintaining the life of infants at high risk of death or severe disability. The key dilemma of neonatal medicine relates to continuing care for patients whose future possibility of survival is extremely uncertain. A large body of literature deals with issues such as appropriate levels of clinical intervention, contesting definitions of future quality of life, and how end-of-life decisions are made or should be made in NICUs.[1] However, these works do not directly attend to the nature of sociality that organizes technological and social relations around newly born human beings in intensive care settings. Sick infants' very dependence on life-sustaining technologies indicates that they are the living embodiment of others' actions, intentions, and obligations.[2] Recovery and growth of the infant patient is not just a physical reaction to intensive treatment: it also "bears witness to the effectiveness of a relationship with" caregivers in the NICU (Strathern 1988, 294).

Paying close attention to the ways in which life-sustaining relations are initiated, lived, and severed in the neonatal ward, I examine how caregiving is realized through a conjunction of engagement and distancing. Two aspects of neonatal medicine have particular importance for understanding the nature of care in this particular setting. One is the very otherness of sick newborns in their liminal phase of life. While in a familiar scenario of socialization the newly born infant is gradually incorporated into caring relations with its mother, father, and kin, joining the realm of belonging, neonatal medicine poses a kind of interruption.[3] It makes life possible for the sickly infant yet prolongs the in-between stage of nativity and fortifies the otherness of the newly arrived human being. Another, equally important aspect is the transient nature of neonatal care. According to its medical definition, twenty-eight days after birth an infant is no longer a neonate

(Kenner and Lott 2013). This does not mean that the patient has to be immediately discharged after this short period, but it implies that this specific organization of care has to be dissolved after a certain time.

While otherness and temporality are mutually implicated in neonatal medicine, caring relations around sick infants always entail the contingency of estrangement. Young human life has to be saved, but doing so may not always be possible or morally defensible. Death, or departure from life, is in fact one acceptable outcome in neonatal care (Vermeulen 2004; Walther 2005), and the pragmatic and skilled ways in which NICU nurses and doctors respond to the need to withhold life-sustaining treatment show that detachment is a fundamental aspect of care and not its negation. Exploring disjunctive connections emerging around sick infants, I argue that organizing care for patient-guests at the threshold between birth and death is not simply motivated by a limitless commitment to sustaining biological life. Instead it involves the unexpected potential of extremely young human beings to elicit relations of care and the relational work that is subsequently required for them.

In the following, I briefly discuss the changing biopolitical landscape of reproductive technology in Chiang Mai that has integrated neonatal care into the service of the state. Then, with a focus on the narratives, affect, and materiality of the deaths of two patients, I demonstrate how life-sustaining factors such as kinship, biomedical treatment, and bureaucratic identification are initiated, disintegrated, and transformed in the process of neonatal intensive care.

Local Morbidity from Premature Births

As I briefly discussed in chapter 1, Ban Phaet Hospital NICU, which came about as an active response to the chronic shortage of NICU beds in Chiang Mai, has become an important node for neonatal care in the region. Through the public hospital networks and referral center, newborn patients from all around Chiang Mai and Mae Hong Son provinces are transferred to Ban Phaet Hospital NICU. After a year's preparation, this NICU opened in 2006 with one pediatrician and five nurses, and by 2008, the number of staff had increased to two pediatricians and ten nurses and nurses' aides with varying degrees of training. The NICU also came equipped with ventilators, incubators, blood gas analyzers, and other testing machines that allowed this ward to operate independently. From October 2007 to December 2010, it treated 286 patients with a variety of symptoms and body weights.

Along the continuum of universal antenatal care and hospital delivery care, neonatal medicine has started to become a normative part of reproductive health care in Chiang Mai. The total number of beds for newborn patients is still not enough for the area's total population, but establishing the NICU in the district hospital has been part of a significant public health effort to make neonatal care widely accessible and available. In a situation where hospital births are becoming increasingly common even in remote rural areas, the public hospital network has efficiently transferred premature and sick newborn babies to the network of NICUs. It also signals the changing topography of biopolitics: neonatal care has been recast as a service of the state, and sick newborn babies have become a legitimate and desirable subject of state-sponsored biomedical intervention.

As this emerging mission of public health care has made a life-and-death difference for numerous newborns, neonatal death also has taken a medicalized form. Many critically sick babies from all around Chiang Mai province are given the chance to receive intensive care, but some of them wind up dying far from home. In May 2012, a dying baby whose flesh was already being eaten by maggots was admitted to Ban Phaet Hospital's NICU. The baby girl had been found by a villager who was picking mushrooms in the forest and who took her to the local district hospital emergency room. The infant was then promptly transported by ambulance around three hundred kilometers to Ban Phaet Hospital and connected to a ventilator. She lived only three hours more in the NICU, but the whole public health system had backed her very short survival. The newly drawn baseline is that the public health system cannot deny biomedical care to a sick newborn.

The second important aspect of neonatal medicine in Ban Phaet Hospital is that there is a significant correlation between premature birth and stratified citizenship. Internal statistics show how this ward has provided essential neonatal care to marginalized non-Thai and migrant populations. According to the NICU patient registration record from November 2011 to September 2012, 64 percent of the total number of patients were covered by universal health coverage for Thai citizens, while 20 percent were covered by Compulsory Migrant Health Insurance, and 16 percent of them were uninsured. In terms of ethnic categories, only 37.5 percent of all patients were Thai, and the rest were Shan and other ethnic minorities. These patterns in neonatal patient admission are connected to families' socioeconomic status. From 2007 to 2012, only one patient was covered by the Civil Servant Medical Benefit Scheme—which insures a segment of the middle- and upper-middle-class population—while the number of uninsured patients, mainly those whose mothers were undocumented migrants, ethnic minorities, and refugees, had steadily increased. The NICU staff also shared the view that premature birth, especially premature birth by non-Thai women, was a result of economic hardship, rural and urban discrepancies in health service distribution, and insecurity related to migration and lack of citizenship.

Neonatal intensive care is the most expensive medical intervention available in Ban Phaet Hospital, yet medical staff do not triage care according to patients' insurance status. On their admission to the ward, uninsured patients, mostly the children of undocumented migrants and refugees, are offered the same intensive care and high-cost medications as insured patients. As this NICU's openness contributes to friction over the broader biopolitical regime that legitimizes the exclusion of noncitizens from public health care, it offers an interesting opportunity to understand the relationship between responsibility and otherness in stepping aside from the thanatopolitics of sovereignty. In this NICU, care is unconditionally distributed in a sense that medical staff always initiate life-sustaining relations for newborn patients upon their arrival. Here, I do not argue that this specific organization of neonatal care is unaffected by broader political processes of producing differentiated legitimacy and inequality of human lives.[4] Rather, I want to emphasize that the major task that is given to the NICU staff is not defining eligible and qualified subjects of care but rather creating a space of belonging for these fragile others. A closer look at how strands of relations are assembled and fail to sustain around a critically sick newborn will help us understand the generative force of elicitation.

The Dying Baby and the Relational Force of Neonatal Medicine

On December 22, 2010, Suthep, a 1.522-kilogram baby boy, was born prematurely at thirty-two weeks gestational age after a failed abortion attempt.[5] Severe birth asphyxia, cardiac arrest, and severe respiratory distress syndrome marked just the beginning of his turbulent life. After resuscitation, the baby also suffered from several infections and metabolic imbalance. On his fifth day after admission to the NICU, his mother, Plae, a twenty-eight-year-old Thai woman, left the ward without a word. Plae told other NICU mothers that she was going out to buy some snacks, but she did not return. Three days later, Plae called me and explained that she had gone out to find the baby's father and, as soon as she found him, she would return.

On January 14, after twenty-three days of intensive therapy, Suthep was finally weaned off the ventilator. This was good news, but he soon developed excessive cerebrospinal fluid in his brain. His head's circumference increased 2.5 centimeters in a week, while his weight gain was very slow. On January 22, Plae finally returned to the hospital with a man who, she insisted, was Suthep's father. Leon, a twenty-five-year-old Thai man, a construction worker, was not quite sure that the baby was his own. Plae had not told him anything when she was pregnant, and they had been out of touch for many months. Dr. Phong expressed his concern about the baby's worsening condition and tried to persuade them that this was a critical time for the parents to be with their baby. Yet Plae refused to stay in the ward, giving the reason that her breast milk already had dried up.

After their short conversation with the doctor, Plae and Leon fought on the veranda of the ward, punching and kicking each other. A nurse had to forcibly separate them. Dr. Phong made no attempt to hide his frustration and bitterness when he told me: "They should understand the serious condition of the baby. No one is standing by him now. What more do I have to say to them? If there is no one left for the baby, it's impossible to help him." He hoped that the baby's grandmother would intervene and take charge. At this point, the NICU staff's request was to register the baby's birth. Without this process, it was extremely difficult to arrange a consultation with specialists at the university hospital. Yet no one wanted to do this for the baby.

As we discussed Suthep's grave condition, Nurse Thip told me several times that there was no reason to feel sad or bitter about the baby. "We can take care of him anyway. And if he survives, I will find a place that the baby can go. I explained to the mother several times that birth registration does not mean that she has to raise the baby herself, but she doesn't understand what really goes on here. That's all. She is just confused and cannot think straight. But we will do what we can for the baby." As Thip predicted, Suthep received full attention from the NICU staff.

On February 3, however, Suthep's condition drastically worsened. At 8 p.m., his oxygen saturation level dropped to 60 percent and his heart rate fell to 50 bpm. Ari, the oldest NICU nurse, in her fifties, gently rubbed the baby's body, disconnected a tube to the ventilator, and did manual ventilation for half an hour. Finally, the baby was stabilized and put back on the ventilator support. At 11 p.m., when Ari changed Suthep's diaper, she made a gentle humming sound to console the baby, who could not cry because of the tube. The soft and calming sound filled the space in the quietness of the late night.

On February 5, Dr. Phong changed the direction of Suthep's treatment to basic care by moving him to the oxygen box. He prescribed no additional medication or further tests. On the following day, when I was having a conversation with Dr. Phong, Leon, Suthep's presumed father, came into the ward with his mother. Dr. Phong introduced me to Suthep's grandmother as a Korean PhD student doing research in the NICU, and he explained the baby's grave condition. Contrary to Dr. Phong's hope, the presumed grandmother did not want to be involved and proposed sending Suthep to the orphanage. In response to her request, Dr. Phong explained again that the condition of the baby's lungs was very grave and his head was filled with water. Then Dr. Phong asked the grandmother what she wanted him to do for the baby in his final moments. The grandmother answered briefly, "It's up to the doctor." Dr. Phong asked her again whether she wanted him to do CPR for the baby if he stopped breathing. She replied, "When the time comes, then he should go." Informed consent for a do-not-resuscitate order was made without any paperwork.

After Suthep was detached from the ventilator, the nurses continued to care for him: regular feeding, a gentle morning bath, and monitoring of his vital signs. Yet although some medications were still provided, the doctor's daily order for him had been minimized: no more extra tests were requested. Dr. Phong once told me that he did not expect that Suthep could survive for such a long time with no mechanical respiratory support, saying, "The baby is really tenacious, isn't he?" Dr. Phong had originally planned to send the baby to the university hospital as soon as he stabilized enough for further treatment, yet in his current condition this plan would not work.

In the oxygen box, the baby did not make any noise and lay silently, with no tubes around him. Hong, the young nurse's aide who had bravely stopped Suthep's parents' fight, told me, "The baby cannot go until he has paid all of his karmic debt. We all know there is no hope for the baby. But, after we removed the tube, the baby continued to live. His suffering will continue until he exhausts his karmic debt [*thueng mot wen mot kam*]." Her emphasis on the karmic cycle of life did not mean that Suthep was destined to suffer; rather, she noted that the time for Suthep's death was set by his own karma, and no one could alter this.

And the time came. Suthep had quietly stayed in the oxygen box for five days more and died at 2:37 a.m. on February 10. It was his fifty-first day in the NICU.

End-of-Life Care, Neonatal Personhood, and Karma

In Suthep's short life, there were many failures and shortcomings. His body had failed to enter a normal track of biological growth, and relationships in his family had crumbled. As Plae unexpectedly left the ward, what struck me was the head nurse's calm and decisive acceptance of the situation rather than condemnation of the mother. As she emphasized, once the patient entered the NICU, the obligation of care and protection was primarily on the NICU staff. Here, medical professionals were proactive to encourage maternal bonding and kin relations around the patient, but when this effort failed, they themselves became the only party taking responsibility for the baby's well-being. Dr. Phong hoped that his authoritative intervention would help the formation of kin relations around the patient, but Suthep's presumed kin were not that malleable.

In this liminal phase of human life, the NICU operates as a collective form of the maternal agent that, in Strathern's words, reveals its "enveloping maternity" (1988, 250). As long as Suthep remained in the ward, the NICU had to provide the foundation for his life and death, and the social life of Suthep had mainly emerged through biomedical mediations and prosthetic extensions. The ventilator, cardiac monitor, touches of the nurses, feeding tubes, nursing notes, doctor's orders, birth and death certificates, as well as his karmic ties—all were the elaborations of partial connections that had extended from his fragile body and made his short life possible. These circuits of care, partly effective and dysfunctional and partly mechanical and human (Haraway [1985] 2003), had enabled Suthep's existence.

Suthep's very passivity, as a biological being and a social person who existed only through these circuits of care, had exercised unexpected agency.[6] His fragility and biological unsustainability had compelled others to do something and search for possibilities to engage with him, regardless of his obscure status. Although Suthep's mother was a Thai citizen, without birth registration he shared several commonalities with the "undeserving" and "illegitimate" patients who sought care from this hospital: he was like an "illegal migrant" with no formal status, papers, and identification. But regardless of this lack of documentation, Suthep had been among the patients with a legitimate claim to the expensive medications, human resources for intensive care, and scarce ventilator support he had received. For Suthep, biomedicine had become an anarchic expenditure of hospitality that was poured into the immediate continuance of his biological trajectory.

Suthep's very short life crystallizes a core issue of social relations mediated by biomedicine: the assemblage of care that once made Suthep's life possible also facilitates his death through technological and affective engagement and distance. Clarifying some preconditions of Suthep's personhood helps us understand this disjunctive interplay of contact and separation. In the process of providing care to Suthep, medical professionals were not very concerned about whether he was conscious or not. Surely, they were interested in the neurological signs and interactive cues he showed, but the general consensus was that the integrity of consciousness did not define his personhood. Unlike a comatose patient, a critically sick neonate does not have a previous identity and memory to recover. All newly born babies are indeed "incomplete persons" (Kaufman 2003, 2260) to a greater and lesser degree according to their level of development. Moreover, the general idea of personhood in Thailand is not to be separated from the notion of karma.[7] In the course of care, Suthep's karmic debt appeared as an independent force that could define the span of his life. It was impossible to know how much pain he had experienced because of the clinical interventions, but he suffered as do all other human beings.

When Suthep's condition worsened, the law of karma appears to be a guiding principle of how to engage with him, although his family members and medical staff applied this principle in a different way. For his family members, the matter of his life and death was not something that they wanted to be involved in; it had to be determined by his own fate. For the NICU staff, although they reached a clinical impasse when there was no available treatment for making changes in Suthep's deteriorating condition, their responsibility for him remained the same as before. Only their care plan had to be changed to allow his death to occur. Withdrawal of life-sustaining care was realized in a passive and gentle manner. He was moved from the ventilator to the oxygen box; several tests were omitted; and no more treatment orders were given for him. But this changing pattern of engagement was not regarded as a way to hasten his death. As the nurse's aide eloquently said, the baby would remain under her care until his destined time for death arrived.

The oddity embedded in this passive approach to the withdrawal of life-sustaining care is that although Suthep's life was totally dependent on care from others, the people who had ministered his life process expressed their own incapacity by invoking Suthep's own fate. In this NICU, medical professionals shared the idea that withdrawal of life-sustaining care was not something they could choose or execute. This moral positioning is surely related to broader Buddhist ethics. Discussing common objections to euthanasia in the arena of Buddhist medical ethics, Damien Keown notes that, in the vein of canonical teachings that emphasize profound respect for life, "death is neither intended nor chosen as either a means or an end" (1995, 63; see also Stonington 2012). Yet I want to emphasize that neonatal medicine's complicated ethical and practical role of administering death is deeply situated in the process of the relational transition from involvement to detachment. It is not simply determined by a general Buddhist moral disposition. When I asked Dr. Phong how long Suthep would be in the NICU, his answer was, "It is not something we can decide. It might be worthless to take care of him this long, but if he tries to live, we should let him live." By disclaiming his ability to make a decision as a doctor, Dr. Phong carefully conferred power to Suthep's chaotic life. In doing so, he limited his involvement and acknowledged that caring relations around the dying baby had been strained.

The NICU staff had tried several clinical and nonclinical interventions to assert relational connections around Suthep, but their aim was not to make him live against limits. Neonatal medicine had worked as a relational medium, but within its double movement, it also had to be disconnecting and separative. The flourishing intimacy and care toward the critically sick baby necessitated careful detachment. In the process of end-of-life care, karma was invoked not as a final explanation of the patient's fatal condition but as a way to facilitate relational separation. The moment of neonatal death provides a window into how neonatal medicine operates as a willful enactment of involvement and separation. Let me turn to the last moments of the baby in bed no. 1, whom we met briefly in the beginning of this chapter.

Nurses' Tactile Engagement with Death

On June 6, 2010, the condition of the baby in bed no. 1 had worsened, and the hospital staff were still unable to contact his mother. After nine days of intensive respiratory therapy, Dr. Samohn finally wrote "NR (No Resuscitation)" on the baby's daily chart. On June 7, around 8:30 p.m., the cardiac monitor connected to the bed was beeping unceasingly, signaling that the baby was in critical condition. There were no more daily orders from the doctor in the baby's chart. The last dose of IV fluid ended, and Nurse Nim muted the cardiac monitor and checked the baby's body temperature again. Then, Nurse Nim put a soft blanket over the baby's belly and increased the temperature of the radiant warmer to give him more warmth. She flashed the penlight at the baby's eye and explained to me that there was no pupillary reflex. Nurse Nim checked and recorded the baby's vital signs on the chart, but this time she did not give him any more chest massages with an electric toothbrush. The baby was still connected to the ventilator, but his blood gas levels and oxygen saturation had not been monitored since the day before. Without the test results, it was impossible to know whether his oxygen demand was being properly met. When I asked what more the doctors could do for him, Kaet, a thirty-two-year-old nurse, said to me that the baby needed his mother, not the treatment. When I asked Nurse Nim about the condition of the baby, she told me, "He may not make it until tomorrow morning." The vital signs of the baby had fluctuated while he remained in critical condition. That night I was unsure whether it would be better to remain in the NICU and await the moment of death or go home. Then Thip, the head nurse, invited me to stay during her shift, which would end at midnight.

The night feeding was done, and I was sitting near the nurses' station and chatting with them. Thip taught me how to sing the legendary folk song "Chiang Mai Girl," and my rendition brought gales of laughter from the nurses and mothers in the ward. The nurses looked tired, but all tried to maintain some degree of cheerfulness. After a short break, the nurses were busy writing notes in the patients' charts. At 9:30 p.m., Nurse Kaet turned off the muted monitor of bed no. 1 and disconnected the tube linking the ventilator and the endotracheal tube inserted into the baby's windpipe for a short while. Then, she checked the baby's heartbeat with a stethoscope. It only took a couple of minutes. Next, Nurse Kaet reconnected the tube to the ventilator and lowered the ventilator setting. Because the baby could not breathe without respiratory assistance, the lower setting would eventually end his breathing. Nurse Kaet listened to the baby's heartbeat again and repeated the procedure one more time.

Just before 10 p.m., Nurse Kaet pronounced the time of death, and Nurse Nim called Dr. Samohn to report it. Nurse Kaet took off the cotton pads shading the baby's eyes from the light of the radiant warmer. The baby's eyes were open. As Nurse Kaet took out the tube from the baby's mouth, his lips were blue. Nurse Nim closed his eyes, applied baby powder on the body, and put him in new clothes. She again covered the baby with a new sky-blue cotton blanket. Then she put the baby's body into an orange plastic bag and put on the label the baby's name that was given to him by the nurse for his birth certificate. As the dead body was left alone on his bed, the monitor connected to bed no. 6 started beeping. Nurse Nim urgently reported the blood test result to Dr. Samohn on the phone and prepared an extra blood pack for the struggling baby. At 11:30 p.m., the night shift nurses arrived in the NICU and started a change-of-shift report with evening shift nurses. Nurse Nim sorted out the documents for the death registration of the baby in bed no. 1 and told the other nurse that the "passport to heaven [*phatsapot pai thi sawan*]" had not yet been filled in.

~

As I described briefly in the beginning of this chapter, from the start every available treatment from this NICU had been given to the patient in bed no. 1, the son of an undocumented Shan migrant. His hospital bills climbed to more than 50,000 baht (around USD 1,490), but the termination of treatment had nothing to do with the treatment cost and his uninsured status. Dr. Samohn wrote the no resuscitation order based on the baby's deteriorating physical condition: she had tried to treat his persistent pulmonary hypertension for several days, but his lungs failed to start their normal function. And it became clear that the baby could not be weaned from the mechanical ventilator. The absence of any pupillary reflex could have indicated brain death, but in this blurred boundary between life and death, making the diagnosis of brain death was not the utmost consideration.

That night, the nurses' acts of care eventually demarcated the boundary between life and death. What the nurses did that night was a rite of *ploi* (letting go), or allowing the patient to leave.[8] As in the case of Suthep when the available treatment turned out to be futile, all the medical professionals could do in this NICU was to allow the sick newborn to live as long as it could, releasing it to die when the time came. The concept of *ploi* conveys both letting live and allowing to die. In the case of the baby in bed no. 1, the "no resuscitation" order did not mean that the medical professionals formally decided to terminate care for the patient. Rather, caring continued within the continuum of dying and death. Although the doctor did not give any specific order for the patient, the nurses kept checking vital signs and recording the baby's movements while providing warmth. When the nurse put cream on the baby's eyelids, there was no hope for a dramatic recovery, but caring attention did not cease.

In this context, note that the doctor did not direct the nurse's actions. No one had given the order to lower the ventilator setting and separate the baby temporarily from the ventilator. No one had directly asked Nurse Kaet, the nurse who finally pronounced the death of the baby, to undertake these procedures. Indeed, the nurse's actions had given a gentle nudge to the process of dying. As we witnessed, the nurses did not explicitly discuss the death process with their colleagues, but they included this passage into death in the flows of their mundane caring practices. As they changed the diaper for the baby, as they measured the amount of milk for feeding, the nurses sought potential avenues of inviting death. Again, it would be inaccurate to describe this moment as one in which a choice or decision was being made to let the baby die. The nurse's actions did not result from discursive negotiations assessing the value or social worth of giving care to this dying patient. Rather, they continued to give care as long as the fragile patient's body allowed them to.

The nurses' actions as death drew near were partly intentional and partly spontaneous: the baby could possibly have survived the night and lived one more day, and if the parents had been on their way to see their child, the nurses would certainly have done their best to keep the baby alive one more day. But the mother never answered the phone, and the nursery had become busy with new patients. I do not imply that the nurse made an economic decision to maximize the use of the NICU facilities. Instead, within the contingency of the ward situation, such as the number of total patients, the graveness of the patient's condition, and the baby's family situation, the NICU nurses were attuned to the moment in an undetermined way. Separating the baby from the ventilator for a short time might hasten the death of the baby, but at that moment the nurse's action was intuitive rather than calculative. The art of caregiving that the nurses presented was fluid, neither forcing the ending nor resisting the limits of life.[9]

The final stage of care reveals the quality of the social contacts that have formed between the nurses and the dying baby. The nurses were very closely involved in the baby's life, but they also had to simultaneously detach themselves from him. Caring relations in the NICU are temporary and two-sided in a most respectful sense: they entail the conjoining of intimate involvement and impersonal detachment.[10] At birth, the newborn baby has been incorporated into the social world through the mediation of neonatal medicine, but in the passage to death, these intense and primary ties must be severed. In the patient's transition out of the NICU, separation through death is a central facet of care, and the nurses work as skillful "practitioners of relational detachment" (Candea 2010, 255).

After Death: The Power of Being There Together

For the NICU staff, neonatal death is distressing, but it also contains something hopeful, as indicated by the name the nurses use for the death certificate, "the passport to heaven." Death signifies that the baby is on the way to rebirth and that its pain and suffering have ended. After a baby dies, there are still several things left for the nurses to do. The baby in bed no. 1 had no family, so one of the nurses had to go to the district office to register his death. Through this bureaucratized and institutional practice, the very short existence of this obscure alien would become a part of the wider collectivity, the population. Unlike Suthep, whose mother was Thai, this baby of a Shan migrant mother did not have to be sent to the public mortuary. Nonetheless, the dead body had to be sent somewhere. The NICU has an informal arrangement with the local temple such that if the parents do not want to take the dead bodies of their children, the bodies are directed to the temple. Most parents were not willing to take their dead children home, so many NICU patients were buried in the small yard of the local temple. The morning after the death of the patient in bed number 1, the head nurse made a call to the temple, and now he was to be buried at the temple.[11] All these arrangements that must be made after death indicate the scope of the NICU nurses' duties: they facilitate not only life but also in some cases death.

This practical engagement with many forms of life—being newly born, dying, being alive, and being dead—is not something peculiar or heroic, but it is commonly found in Chiang Mai at several moments of the transitions in life. When the nurses put the dead baby in the paper box to send him to the temple, they also put in some new clothes and baby blankets as an offering made for the spirit of the baby. And the head nurse also prepared a small amount of money to send the temple: there would be no special funeral service for the dead baby, but the money would be used to make merit for his spirit. The nurses made these small caring gestures toward the baby's spirit, as people usually did for the funerals of their family members, friends, and neighbors. The basic logic of making merit for the other is that the living aid the dead. By giving offerings, the dead are invited as consociates of the living, the ghost as stranger is welcomed, and the strings between them are reconfirmed.[12] As we have also observed in the NICU, invoking the unknown other's presence and being present to the other's needs are grounds for making hospitable relations of care.

Enacting Hospitality

The increased access to neonatal intensive care in Chiang Mai signals how the health of infants has become a critical object of biopolitical intervention, especially when the ideal of universal coverage is seriously pursued. The NICU's openness to newborns with obscure ties to kin or the nation-state reveals the particular legitimacy given to conserving human life in its infancy. Yet this modest NICU exhibits its biomedical effectiveness not only by saving sick newborns from death but also by ritualistically anchoring and incorporating fragile human life into the social world. Sickly newborns' dependence on life-sustaining care reveals that biomedical mediations and technological prosthetic extensions are constitutive of a particular personhood and nurturing work. Here, the practices of neonatal medicine prove to have unusual effectiveness, as they open a relational field in which social others engage each other.

I have proposed to call this relational engagement elicitation, and the NICU staff's commitment to these vulnerable subjects of care sheds light on the moments when the ethics of hospitality comes together with the force of elicitation. The quality of social ties between the attentive but disinterested medical professionals and the critically sick babies in need of care is explained by neither institutionally structured pragmatics nor sympathy for human misery. The nurses and doctors play the nurturer's role, by responding to the presence of these extremely young and defenseless lives.[13] More importantly, such work is not a matter of who has the power to authorize and administer life and death, to make live and let die. The doctors and nurses in Ban Phaet Hospital NICU justify the provision of care based on neither criteria of bureaucratic legitimacy nor technical measures of outcomes of care based on the patient's potential future social worth. Taking responsibility for unknown strangers who are passing through the liminality of birth and life or life and death—being elicited by their changing presence—the nurses and doctors in the NICU hardly question whether they should provide care. Instead they continuously responded to the matter of "how to care" to deal with their biologically and socially fragile charges.

In this domain of "how to care," the life and death of others fall upon the NICU staff.[14] Their embodied practices that are attuned to the immediate needs of others indeed yield a hospitable moment. Of significance is that hospitality in this context is not "a reaction to, or decision about, ethical precepts in given political circumstances" (Humphrey 2012, S63). In this NICU, unconditional openness is an ethical virtue, yet it becomes real only through the relational dynamics of engagement and separation. Thus, care ends after a certain time not as a form of calamitous exclusion but by an enactment of hospitality. This particular mode of sociality also illuminates the notion that distancing is not a simple refusal to acknowledge. Instead it is constitutive of caregiving.[15]

The current infrastructure of neonatal medicine in Chiang Mai is situated within the wider political and economic context of health care provision in which the lives of illegitimate and distant others are unequally valued. Yet the NICU staff's ability to save, nurture, comfort the fragile, and sometimes make death happen unexpectedly reveals the possibility of conceiving relations to the unknown stranger as an integral part of health care and the ethics of biomedicine. Their everyday effort exhibits the productive power of care that emerges when one is compelled to find a way to be together with vulnerable others.

5

Vulnerability and Nurturance at Home

After long and wearisome stays in the hospital, the patients with whom I had been spending time returned home. With their departures, my field site also began to grow as I followed the recovered babies, new and experienced mothers and fathers, and elderly patients from the NICU, wards, and clinics to their homes. As their environments changed, so too did the work of care that was needed. The unfinished homes of Shan migrants on busy urban construction sites and remote agricultural farms were the pronounced nodes where I witnessed people's relentless commitments to health, prosperity, and dignity. In conditions of deprivation, pursuing care often turns out to be injurious, but nevertheless, taking responsibility for care of oneself and others appears to be a way to nurture the possibilities for transformation. In this chapter, I will illuminate politico-economic, physical, and affective vulnerabilities that are especially accentuated after childbirth. As pregnancy and childbirth impose lasting effects on women's lives, enacting the maternal role contains a serious risk and danger especially for those in precarious situations. It may be that the maternal is a "primary instance of *care* for the *other*" (Cavarero 2016, 100) as widely recognized in feminist ethics, yet in migrant women's everyday struggle for survival, it is self-care that turns out to be a critical element in forging motherly care. I further explore how the elicitation of affirmative relations takes central place in women's struggles with self-care and child-rearing.

The encampments of Shan migrant families on construction sites and agricultural farms in Chiang Mai offer a direct example of the calamities that people have to endure when the juxtaposition of wage labor and social reproduction is extremely condensed. People work, eat, sleep, have sex, and raise children within a small radius of the work site, and here the domesticity of the home is encapsulated within the exploitative labor regime. Maintaining households is never meant to be easy in these conditions, which continually give rise to crises of (re)production.[1] The air of tiredness that surrounds Shan migrant women's bodies indicates the double burden of being a wage laborer and a mother. Even if it is a makeshift hut in a shanty town, the home is assumed to be the primary place where the work of birthing and raising the young is done along with the care for sick and elderly family members. For many Shan women in this situation, having such a home and being responsible for the daily needs of care constitute an audacious project that often goes beyond the bounds of possibility.

In this chapter, I tell three Shan women's stories of nurturing the self and the family. During my years of fieldwork, these women were the key figures who pushed me to look beyond biomedical models of illness and consider the stories of the vulnerable people who are in charge of care in the domestic sphere. In the preceding chapter I elaborated how intensive care for critically sick neonates is based on political and ethical aspects of dealing with fundamental human vulnerabilities. Here I look at how nurturers who are under an obligation to care for their young dependents also struggle with their own embodied susceptibility to harm, injury, and abandonment. In the half-demolished homes of Shan migrants, it is evident that deep traces of structural violence make their lives insecure.[2]

Impoverished Shan women's experiences of birth and child-rearing illustrate how the vulnerable must sometimes find convoluted ways of eliciting care for the self and others. Instead of using migrant women's stories as examples of heroic or victimized motherhood, I seek to understand layers of complexity about nurturance particularly during the period following childbirth. The work of care done by these women is deeply embedded in the double burden of domestic and wage labor and is similarly mundane, repetitive, exhausting, and exploitative. Yet what I began to discern in the homes of the women I visited is not the sheer impoverishment of life but something closer to vigorous "world-making projects [emerging from their] practical activities of making lives" (Tsing 2015, 21–22).

Sen, an Ascetic Mother

In the Ban Phaet Hospital female ward, Sen, whom I introduced briefly in chapter 3, was noticeable in her winter outfit. In the middle of a hot summer day—the temperature hit 37 degrees Celsius—she wore a woolen hat, a long-sleeve shirt over her hospital gown, and thick socks. Beads of sweat stood on her nose. A thirty-year-old Shan woman, she had given birth to a healthy, 3.1-kilogram baby boy on May 15, 2010. Sen was devotedly observing *yu duean*, a traditional one-month postpartum practice. In the female ward, it was easy to find several Thai and Shan mothers observing some sort of postpartum regime, including keeping the body warm, maintaining dietary restrictions, and taking herbal medicine. This type of postpartum care is widely observed in Southeast Asia, although the kinds of rules and restrictions vary widely.[3] The common logic of this practice rests on the notion that the first month after birth is considered to be the most vulnerable period for a new mother. To restore strength and allow the mother to "mature" (Hanks 1963), she is required to observe several rules and remain in seclusion.

While I found many variations on postpartum practices in the Ban Phaet Hospital female ward, Sen was the most enthusiastic and diligent exponent I encountered. Wearing warm clothes, Sen ate only the rice porridge from the hospital meals and did not touch any other food. Along with the prescribed drugs, she also took a special herbal medicine to increase the air, or wind (*lom*), in her body.[4] In the ward, nurses were tolerant of most postpartum practices except for bathing restrictions. The head nurse of the female ward explained to me, "We don't ask the patients not to follow *yu duean* rules. We tell them there are many ways of doing this, and taking a warm bath can be good for them. For their convenience, we prepare the electric kettle for drinking water and a water heater in the shower stall." To show her compliance with the nurses' orders, Sen went into the bathroom, but she only washed her body with a wet towel. Sen thought that it was better not to take a shower during the first three days after childbirth.

After her discharge, Sen's postpartum practice continued rigorously at home with her husband's help. Khiaw, her thirty-four-year-old husband, a day laborer working on vegetable plantations, had done all the farm work and laundry for the first month after the birth of their child. When Khiaw went out to work, Sen stayed alone in their little concrete block house on the fringe of the village with her newborn son, keeping several prohibitions. All these efforts were to prevent *lom phit duean* (wind afflictions caused by doing something wrong in the postpartum month), which could affect her health in the long term. Any inappropriate practices or the intake of the wrong food during the postpartum month is thought to cause several symptoms of ill health ranging from general weakness and headaches to partial paralysis, madness, and even death.[5] The symptoms of these afflictions can appear long after the child's birth, so undertaking proper postpartum care is considered important for a women's long-term health and has implications for her future fertility and ability to work. The vulnerability of a new mother is attributed not only to humoral disturbances and physical weakness but also to her susceptibility to malevolent spirits. Sen explained to me that young women, especially those who have just given birth, can be easily affected by evil spirits. For protection, Sen wore on her neck and tied on the wrist of her newborn baby red threads, which she called *lak phoy*, a kind of auspicious amulet.

Dietary restrictions are crucial aspects of postpartum care practices, and Sen was very cautious about not eating food that could possibly cause wind afflictions. As a result, her daily meal became very modest: she would have only rice with a small selection of vegetables such as cabbage and mustard greens. Spices and several common vegetables, including cucumber and eggplant, were thought to bring about negative consequences. Various cooking sauces and ingredients were also restricted: fish sauce, oyster sauce, and all kinds of fermented food were not allowed. She drank only boiled water with dried ginger and no cold drinks. During the postpartum month, I met Sen several times, but I often failed to conform to her dietary rules when I brought her snacks and fruit. For example, dietary restrictions among many northern Thai and Shan women allow grilled pork skewers, but Sen had maintained a strict vegetarian diet since finding out that she was pregnant.

My interest in Sen's practices began when I noted that they differed from existing anthropological observations of this well-known cultural tradition, and I wanted to know more about how Sen arrived at her own judgments regarding her diet during this vulnerable time. Although her regime of meticulous dietary abstinence adhered to the general logic of humoral balance, the question of what she should and should not eat required an ongoing series of judgments.[6] Sen once told me, "When I was in the hospital, they provided such delicious looking food. One day, they served stir-fried cucumbers with oyster sauce and it smelled very nice, but I couldn't eat it. I decided not to eat that one. I saw that several other women who had also given birth ate the food, but I thought that I shouldn't eat cucumber. And oyster sauce was definitely wrong to eat." Sen clearly knew that other Thai and Shan women in the same situation either did not observe any postpartum restrictions or followed different rules from her own.

Multiple criteria of judgment could be applied—her knowledge of how to do *yu duean* is similar to what Bourdieu would call doxa, "the self-evidence of the commensense world" (1977, 167)—but as Sen put her own rules into practice, she had to make her own decisions continuously and stick to them. Being in *yu duean*, observing postpartum restrictions, is both dispositional and performative in the sense that it requires a ritualistic readjustment of everyday conduct.

A possible way of understanding this everyday practice is to see a kind of explanatory model at work in women's experiences of childbirth. Anthropological research on the changing patterns of reproductive health behaviors has focused on the tensions around the modernization and medicalization of childbirth. Anthropologist Andrea Whittaker's (2000) work is a good example of how rural women's insistence on postpartum practices reflects everyday forms of resistance and defiance in the face of biomedical authority. In Sen's case, she clearly recognized the tensions between traditional beliefs and modern biomedical intervention, but her idiosyncratic commitment to postpartum care brought us to another dimension of agency and care-oriented relations. During her pregnancy, she enthusiastically joined every antenatal session and paid close attention to the nurses' advice.

> I understand why the nurses recommended that I eat eggs, fish, and meat. It is all for having a healthy baby, but I decided not to eat meat at all as soon as I knew I was pregnant. My husband needs to eat meat for his strength to work in the fields, and the baby may need to have protein for his good health. I want to make my baby tall, so I might need to feed him some meat. But if possible, I don't want to give any meat to my baby as long as my husband doesn't get upset about this. Anyway I will not feed him buffalo meat. When I was in my hometown, I saw that people killed the buffalo that had worked for us for a long time, and I thought that it was really bad to cause such grave suffering to another life. Eating meat will affect my karma and I would prefer to have more merit by only eating vegetables.

Sen's ruminations on what she should eat suggest that multiple modalities of care can be conjoined in postpartum practices. Rather than resisting the nutritional advice from the hospital, Sen modified her own judgment according to her and others' particular circumstances: everyone in the family had different needs, and Sen anticipated that she would respond differently to their needs and her own. Here, she was neither opposed to biomedical knowledge nor solely reliant on customary scripts. Drawing on multiple modalities of care, Sen instead actively explored the kinds of practices that could work for her at this vulnerable time. Her decision to adopt a vegetarian diet also served to illustrate how eating can become a preventive and exemplary practice. When her concerns turned from nutrition to karma, it became clear to me that her ordinary acts of eating, bathing, and everyday living were construed as protection. And I could understand more about the material changes to her body that these practices had brought about when I visited her home.

A New Mother's Changing Body

When I entered Sen's room a day before the end of her postpartum month, the air was full of smells. The mingling smells of her unwashed body and hair, the herbal medicine, and soured breast milk wafted through the room. Small flies were swarming around Sen and the drops of milk on the floor. Sen turned on the electronic fan for me and my fieldwork collaborator and brought us a bottle of water. Fanning away flies from the sleeping baby, Sen told me, "Khiaw [her husband] forgot to buy vegetables for me to eat, so I just had a bowl of rice with salt." When I asked her what she wanted to eat right now, she smiled at me and replied, "I've badly wanted to have a soup with *chaom* [acasia pennata, green feathery shoots]. But I'm worried that it would be bad for the baby. I should wait five more months until the baby grows up enough."[7] When I asked her again why she followed all these rules, she remarked, "It's a kind of torture that you cannot eat all these things and just watch other people enjoy food. I badly wanted to drink cold water, but it could cause terrible muscle pain four or five years later. Wind affliction is such a scary thing. I know many people who suffer from wind affliction and who have spent lots of money on treating it. So I have to endure this time, because I feel for my baby. If I were to become sick, who would take care of my baby? My parents are not here, and my husband has to go to work; I cannot be sick."

The rather extreme measures Sen was taking testified to her commitment and determination to do what she saw as the best way to care for herself and her baby. No one was forcing her to do this, but she doggedly refrained from eating certain things and bathing, all the while remaining in isolation in the small sweltering room to prevent possible future afflictions that could affect her baby and herself. Leaving the body unwashed so that it becomes enveloped in a strong odor, thus enacting changes to the body through ritualistic daily discipline, is part of the regime Sen followed in an attempt to apply ideas of power and protection in the Theravada Buddhist tradition.[8] A mother's body in *yu duean* (postpartum observance) carries a logic of transformation similar to that of the body of an ascetic forest monk: by enduring bodily discomfort and self-isolation for a significant amount of time, one can acquire protective powers that help to ward off malicious spirits, afflictions, and adversity.[9] Hanks's (1963) classic ethnography on maternity rituals in the Thai context confirms this theme of self-formation: the experience of suffering and endurance during the postpartum month makes the mother more enlightened and compassionate. While an influential study of Shan Buddhism by Nicola Tannenbaum (1995) does not put much emphasis on postpartum rituals, the author makes a broader argument that the practices of restraint and withdrawal are key components for acquiring power and protection.

Again, although the postpartum observance is based on certain religious and ritualistic conventions, it takes different forms depending on the practitioner. The singularity of Sen's postpartum practice is located within the stream of her particular life experience. I began to realize that the bodily transformation that Sen was committed to achieve was deeply associated with her own sense of urgency to be a strong, capable mother who can afford enough protection to her child. Self-care was a way to elicit this kind of transformation.

That day Sen met my research collaborator, Aur, a single woman and graduate student from Chiang Mai University, for the first time. Sen was surprised that Aur was four years older than she was but still looked quite young. Sen told us, "People like me get old quickly. I got married when I was very young and have given birth three times already. And I think too much. Sometimes I can't fall asleep because I worry too much. It makes me get old." Then, she explained to us how her two children had died at a very early age. A thirty-year-old Shan woman, Sen had married three times and given birth three times. Her first marriage in Shan State was arranged by her father when she was in her late teens. Since her father had only daughters, he hoped that his new son-in-law would help with his agricultural work. However, Sen's first marriage did not work out. Her first husband often skipped out on the daily agricultural work, and arguments and quarrels in the family were never ending. After a two-year marriage, Sen divorced her first husband; her father gave him a half share of the rice harvest of that year as compensation.

She then met a solider in the Shan State Army. "He was a really good man and handsome," Sen recalled of the most beloved man in her life. Her parents strongly disapproved of Sen's choice, but she left her hometown and followed her husband for four years in the jungle. "Life in the jungle was really tough. We had to hide from the Burmese soldiers all the time, and we were never properly fed. In the jungle, there was nothing to eat. Sometimes we ate only bamboo shoots for many days. When it rains in the jungle, you even cannot imagine the life there," she told me.

Her first baby was born in the jungle and died shortly after birth. "There was no traditional birth attendant and I had to give birth all alone. I couldn't cut the umbilical cord by myself, so my friend cut the cord for me with a bamboo knife. She didn't know how to do it. When she cut the cord, masses of blood came out and didn't stop. If the blood hadn't come out like that, my baby might have survived. The baby didn't cry at all and had no strength to suck the milk. If I could have given birth in a hospital like those in Thailand, the baby would not have died. I held my baby for hours, but he was gone." Another devastating event occurred in her life when her husband was caught by Burmese soldiers. "I don't know how they knew that my husband was a Shan soldier. He wore normal clothes and planned to stay in the village for a while. I couldn't come out when my husband was caught. If they knew that I was the wife of a Shan soldier, they would have killed me for sure." Sen's husband was hanged to death when she was two months pregnant.

After Sen gave birth to her second child, she met Khiaw, her current husband, who had also spent ten years in the Shan State Army. After Khiaw was discharged from the army, he wanted to have a new life in Thailand and asked Sen to go with him. "There was nothing to do in Burma. There was such a bad drought, so it was impossible to grow anything. And I hadn't helped my parents at all since I married my second husband. In Thailand, I could work and send money to my father." Eventually, Sen decided to send her second child to the baby's grandmother and came to Thailand. After a year, the three-year-old boy died. "I cried all day after I heard the news. The baby's grandmother said that the baby had diarrhea, but in Burma, the only hospital is in the city, it's too far," Sen told me.

"My life is just full of suffering and pain. If I could go back to the past, I would just want to be with my parents. When I was young, there was nothing to worry about. I just did what my parents asked me to do, and they took care of me." Turning to me, she said, "You don't have to marry soon. Women's lives are not easy after we are married. You will get pregnant and have to take care of the children. The responsibility of women is full of suffering because we have less merit than men. Why do I have to suffer like this? I want to do more good deeds, want to have more merit." This was Sen's answer when I asked her why she should not eat meat during the postpartum month. Sen emphasized, "My life is already full of suffering. Why do I have to give more pain to others just to eat? Eating meat involves our karma. I don't want to cause pain and suffering to other lives."

~

Here, I weave together several conversations to show how Sen has lived through violence and painful losses. Her story of childbirth and the loss of two of her children evidences the state violence inflicted by Myanmar's authoritarian government, the personal and collective sacrifice around the prolonged military insurgency, the deepened economic dispossession in Shan State, the risks involving unauthorized migration, and gendered inequality. Her social roles and identities have also drastically changed: she went from being a young daughter to becoming the wife of a militant soldier and then joining the ranks of transnational migrant workers.

Sen's first proper postpartum month was indeed a rare and critical moment in her life. Her ascetic practices during this period of time were firmly intended as a means of restoring her strength before returning to the everyday stream of life. Unlike Buddhist monks, Sen was a lay person and mother who had to quickly return to the everyday activities of living, not to withdraw from them. This everyday-oriented asceticism, which takes the form of renunciation for a limited time period, is applied as an effective means of drawing and gathering protective power around her. Although temporary, Sen's ascetic regime serves the purpose of limiting the claims on her life containing the past, and thus reducing her karmic debt and hence the retributive power of the life-destroying forces that had laid waste to her previous family life. The notion of karma appears to be significant for Sen's practice as it allows her to endure her suffering and to envision the possibility of a better future. This improvised regime of self-care serves to allow her to secure her own power of protection and so to intensify her capacity to nurture.

When a month passed, Sen stopped wearing thick clothes, but she had to take herbal baths for another month, avoid drinking cold water for six months, and continue her vegetarian diet. She wanted to have a proper *ap duean* ceremony (the celebration to mark the end of the postpartum month), but she could not afford the expense. Inviting an elderly Shan for a blessing and preparing food for guests would cost too much money. Sen's postpartum practice ended gradually. The future was unknown, but at that time Sen was strong enough to raise her child and again work in the fields.

Nok, an Afflicted Mother

There were many explanations as to why Nok was sick. When I first met Nok in the Ban Phaet Hospital ward, she was anxiously walking around in her bare feet, holding a plastic bag full of baby clothes. She stormed into the nurses' station and demanded to know when she could go home. The attending nurse told her that her daughter still had a fever, so she had to wait until the doctor came to order her discharge. Nok returned to her bed without replying and shortly afterward returned to the nurses' station. This time she asked for milk for her baby. The nurse was irritated by Nok's rude manner but gave her two packets of soy milk. When I asked the nurse what was going on, she told me that Nok was anxious because she had run out of her medication. "She is just mentally unstable, but she is quite chatty, so if you want, you can talk to her," the nurse told me before introducing me to Nok, beginning a series of encounters.

That day Nok told me that she suffered from *lom phit duean*. When it struck her, she became lethargic and could not breathe. Two days before, she had experienced strong symptoms and called an ambulance to take her to Ban Phaet Hospital with her two-year-old daughter. Nok was the primary patient when she arrived at the hospital, but the doctor noticed that her daughter had a high fever and ordered that she be hospitalized as well. In our first conversation, Nok was eager to talk to me and did not mind other patients listening to our conversation. Nok noticed that my Thai was as clumsy as hers and mimicked my wrong tone with an endearing smile. When I asked what had caused her wind illness, she told me an unexpected story. "I accidentally met my brother in the market next to the big hospital. I hadn't seen him for a long time since I left my hometown in Burma, and he said that our parents had died several years ago. I was so shocked and saddened, so I couldn't do anything. Then, I become *phi ba* [a mad person] and stayed in a psychiatric hospital for a month." The grief at having lost her parents was added to the etiology of her sickness.

Nok had come to Chiang Mai around ten years ago from Shan State. Her age was uncertain, as were many other aspects about her. At our first encounter she told me she was thirty-six, but her hospital bed sign indicated that she was twenty-seven. She also told me that she had worked as a domestic worker and married a Shan man when she was in her early twenties. This first marriage went badly because her husband beat her when he was drunk. "He used to smash my head on the ground. He hit me so badly that I became very weak and sick." Nok then met her current husband, Deng, a Thai born in Chiang Mai, who was working as a night guard at the construction site where Nok had lived. Deng felt sorry for Nok's situation and eventually asked her to leave the construction site with him. After Nok started to live with Deng, she stopped going to work and stayed in Deng's deceased mother's small wooden house in a rural village located around forty kilometers away from Ban Phaet Hospital.

Shortly after moving in with Deng, Nok became pregnant but eventually lost the child through miscarriage. Whereas Nok put little emphasis on her miscarriage, Deng insisted on the linkage between Nok's ill health and her pregnancy. When I met Deng in his house, he explained to me that Nok did not take care of herself during and after her first pregnancy and ate everything without caution: in other words, he insinuated that Nok's carelessness had caused her wind afflictions. Deng also believed that the soul of the dead baby had impacted them: the baby might be angry with them or still want to be with them, and the miscarriage must be connected to their karma. When I asked Deng whether they had tried to get help from local healers or monks, he told me, "They can make up anything to get money from us, right? It's just a wind afflicting illness; they cannot help with these problems." Eventually, Nok had two more children, and after her second delivery, she had a tubal ligation for birth control. While Deng was telling me these things on a bench under an old tilted house, Nok was sitting close to us, but she did not make any comment and kept washing her children's clothes.

Exactly when Nok's nervous breakdown began to occur was unclear. Nok once said that she had felt depressed and lethargic after the miscarriage. Deng remembered that Nok had had a seizure a year after their son was born. In 2010 Nok was a frequent visitor of Ban Phaet Hospital. Her outpatient file was an inch thick, with records of her repeated visits to the outpatient clinic, emergency room, and ward. Nok was also uninsured and had been unable to pay her hospital bills on several occasions. The nurses knew quite well about Nok's situation, but in many cases there was nothing much they could do for her. Her first long-term hospitalization in the psychiatric hospital had happened just a month before we first met. Nok described her time in the psychiatric hospital as comfortable: she spent most of the time there lying down and sleeping. After she had been discharged, Nok continued to take her psychiatric medication. I did not have a chance to accompany her to the psychiatric hospital and could not find out about the diagnosis given to her. Instead, she showed me her daily medications, which were mainly for controlling the symptoms of schizophrenia-like psychosis and epilepsy (trihexyphenidyl, risperidone, and sodium valproate). Nok told me that the drugs made her sleep heavily. For instance, she would be unable to hear the baby's crying and would not wake up until morning.

Nok's claim of wind affliction illness, a specific example of somatization, intrigued me, but each consecutive conversation felt like slipping into murky water as the situation was much more complex than I had initially assumed. Her ill health was attributed to multiple, seemingly incompatible causes: afflicting wind illness brought on by doing something wrong in the postpartum month, the deep sorrow of losing her parents, hyperventilation, the trauma of domestic violence, the wandering soul of the aborted child, and the onset of schizophrenia-like psychosis. The family was destitute and in a chronic state of crisis, and Nok and her children were not well.

In February 2011, the last month of my first round of fieldwork, I visited Nok's house to say good-bye. It was a weekday, but unexpectedly Deng remained in the house to look after his feverish daughter. Urging me to find Seoul on Google Maps with his cheap smart phone, Deng told me that he planned to go to Bangkok to work. I was surprised at his new plan and asked him how he planned to take Nok and his children to Bangkok. Deng had once denied that Nok was a Shan migrant because he was concerned about her undocumented status. This time, however, he was quite open about this issue: "I have already made up my mind. I don't know what will happen in the future, but I might send my children to the orphanage. If Nok is caught by the police, they would send her back to Burma. I don't know." I could not hide my shock at Deng's new plan. In my several interviews with Nok, she had insisted that she had completely forgotten the Shan language and could not even remember where her hometown was. Nok also insisted that she had already lost contact with her siblings in Chiang Mai. What would happen if Deng abandoned her? Every time Nok went to the hospital, she took with her a piece of cardboard paper with Deng's phone number and the emergency number for the ambulance. My contact number was scribbled on the paper too, but she rarely called me. While her husband was telling me of his plan to run away to Bangkok, Nok was calming her crying daughter with a piggyback ride and acting as if she was not listening to us. All the while her closest relation was announcing his possible abandonment of her, and I had no means of intervening on her behalf.

A year later, I returned to Ban Phaet Hospital for my second period of fieldwork and asked the female ward nurses about Nok. They remembered her well and told me that she had been in the ward a month earlier because she had attempted suicide. The nurses were told that Nok had drunk poisin in an attempt to kill herself, but fortunately her condition was not severe. "She was calling for attention, that's all." The nurses reassured me that Nok had not seriously injured herself and was eventually referred to the psychiatric hospital. Before I went to visit Nok's house, I unexpectedly met a caretaker from the health station in Nok's village. She remembered me, the Korean student who had visited Nok several times before, and broke more sad news: Nok had been sexually assaulted by a neighbor and had caused a scene by threatening to commit suicide in her house. I called Deng, Nok's husband, and fortunately he was still in Chiang Mai with Nok.

When I arrived at Nok's house at around midday, the fringe of the village was quiet. From outside the house I could hear that Nok was watching TV with her son. She was surprised to see me again and excitedly invited me to go to the noodle shop together for lunch. The owner of the shop occasionally took care of Nok's children when Nok was in the hospital. As she was fixing noodles for us, the middle-aged lady told me, "It's a good thing that her daughter was sent to the orphanage. The mother cannot take care of her children anyway. See, this boy should be going to school, but still he stays home all day and can't even speak properly." I realized that that was the reason I had not seen Nok's youngest daughter in the house. Listening to the chimes from the elementary school, the three of us ate noodles.

On the way back home, Nok took me to the house of her husband's aunt. The old lady welcomed us and said that Deng hardly comes back home because he has to work all day and night in the city. The old lady told me, "Nok can't do any hard work. She had a seizure before, so she can't work in the fields. She barely manages to clean and cook for the children. Today she has already borrowed 40 baht from me. Her husband gives her money, but she just spends the money on this and that, buying food and sweets for the children. She doesn't know how to save money. She has been like this for a long time, so what we can do?" After a brief chat I left the aunt's house with Nok and her son.

In Nok's ramshackle house we talked a little bit more, and I asked about her daughter. Nok explained that she had been in the psychiatric hospital for two months, and that her husband had sent their two children to the orphanage during that time. The orphanage did not allow her son to stay longer because of his disability. I remembered that Deng had once told me that their first son was diagnosed as "autistic" when he was three. He had registered his son for a government disability subsidy and received 500 baht every month. I knew that Nok and Deng had talked about sending their children to someone—Nok had once suggested that if I wanted she would give me her daughter—but I did not expect that it would actually happen. She said, "I want to send my children to school, but I don't have money. They don't have to live like this with me; it's good for her to be in the orphanage."

I then asked her why she had had to go to the psychiatric hospital the last time, and she briefly told me about the incident. She had gone to an old man's house to give him a massage—Nok used to give massages to old people in her neighborhood, and for this she earned a small amount of money—and he attacked her while her son was watching. "He was really violent and hurt me." A few days after the assault, she took all her medication in one go. After that she was sent to the psychiatric hospital. "Why didn't Deng call the police?" I asked. She answered without outward signs of agitation, "Deng wanted to call the police. But I was ashamed. And when I came back from the hospital, it had already been two months since he did it to me." I could not ask anything more about the sexual assault, but I did want to know how the hospital had responded to her. "What did the doctor say at this time?" I asked her. "That it's just about *lom phit duean* [the wind afflicting illness] and *suemsao* [depression]. Staying in the hospital was good. I took the medicine and fell asleep. They gave me food, and I didn't have to think about any bad things."

Although Nok told me that she felt better after the hospitalization and medication, I wondered about the impact of taking psychiatric medications over several years without being regularly monitored. She had not been offered any regular consultations or checkups from any of the hospitals she had visited. As she explained to me, at the psychiatric hospital she had been prescribed medications not just for neurological problems (*ya prasat*) but also for protection (*ya khumkhrohng*). Nok accepted the different sets of etiologies given to her. In her explanation, wind affliction and depression coexisted without tension, and these two different conceptualizations all together allowed Nok to express her symptoms. What was at stake for her was not so much about figuring out the cause of her ill health but addressing her need for help out loud. As an afflicted person, what mattered to her most was care and protection.

Considering Nok's regular visits, the staff of Ban Phaet Hospital might have been more proactive in her case, yet during my fieldwork I rarely saw home visits organized for patients who suffered from mental health problems.[10] Since Nok had been labeled a psychiatric patient, she was regarded as someone who could only be helped with psychiatric medications. Upon returning to the hospital, I asked the ward nurses if there were any legal procedures that could help rape victims. The nurses' answer was simple: until the patient completes a formal police report, there is nothing that the hospital can do for them. During the rest of my stay in 2012, Nok did not call the ambulance as often as she had before and did not stay overnight in the hospital, even though she sometimes told me that she still heard scary voices in her head. Nok continued to go frequently to the health station in her village, but having grown tired of Nok's repeated visits, the health station staff had stopped keeping records of her outpatient visits long ago. The nurse in the health station told me, "She is not normal [*mai tem*]. She just wants some attention." Once Nok's requests for help and care became trivialized in this way, the primary health care service ceased to be of much assistance.

In the last month of my second fieldwork trip, in 2012, I visited Nok to tell her that I would be going back to Seoul at the end of the week. I asked her if there was anything I could do for her, and she requested some money to recharge her cellphone credit. We went to the shop together, and she called Deng to let him know about my departure. Then, she insisted on walking with me to the village health station where I had parked my car. She entered the health station first and told the nurse that her foot hurt. The caretaker of the health station gave her a small bandage for the scratches on her foot. When we came out to the parking lot, she suddenly said to me, "What he did to me was wrong, right?" "Yes, yes. You didn't do anything wrong. The man was the bad person," I answered precipitously. Then, Nok looked into my eyes, "It's not a big deal anymore. It happened long ago. It's okay, right?" I repeated what she said, "Yes, *mai pen rai*," and hugged her briefly. I felt Nok's hands lightly clutching my back and the warmth of her body around me. When I got into the car, Nok cheerfully said to me, "*Susu!*" while pumping her fist into the air as she had seen in Korean soap operas.[11]

~

It is not my intent to redefine Nok's self-diagnosis of wind illness as a psychiatric crisis. She experienced a breakdown not only of her humoral balance, spirit, and mind and body but also of social relations with those around her, and a long series of afflictions that she had experienced lays bare the traumatic nature of being vulnerable. In her life trajectory, consisting of migration, personal tragedy, domestic violence, and several nervous breakdowns, she had been uprooted from her original Shan kinship ties and relied solely on Thai neighbors and relatives on her husband's side. When Nok insisted that she had forgotten her mother tongue, she might have been trying to turn her focus away from her state of dislocation by expressing her will to belong to the Thai society in which she currently found herself. However, her new Thai husband, kin, and neighbors appear to be distant and even to pose a threat of abandonment to her.

The district hospital and health station may have been among the few places where she felt welcomed and protected. The continued medication and hospitalization during her time of crisis offered a short period of relief, but, in most cases, this remedy failed to acknowledge and engage with the underlying problems that had brought about Nok's highly vulnerable position. The sexual assault incident painfully attested to Nok's fatal precariousness relating to her lack of social and legal protections. The crime was unjustly treated as her individual ills, and eventually, not the rapist but the victim was "locked up," albeit in a psychiatric ward where she found respite from her violent life. The sheer failure of care that happened in these trusted places was that her pain and suffering were either trivialized or treated as uncontrollable except by psychiatric confinement and medication.

Despite all these disappointments and shortcomings, Nok continued to seek help. For two whole years, she had lived in the same place, continued to visit the same health station and asked for medical attention, called the ambulance again and again to take her to Ban Phaet Hospital, all while raising her children by herself. In a way, the nurses were right: Nok was "calling for attention." The vital importance lies in her insistent demand for recognition and care; by doing so, she made her social existence present. As a migrant woman who is deeply marginalized and afflicted, Nok's social presence would be easily rendered nothing. Yet she did not let it happen. Just as Veena Das (2010) has noted in her contemplation of the convergence of violence and the everyday, Nok's troubled, demanding presence in this local landscape could itself be seen as an achievement, however fragile and temporary. Trying to stay within the bounds of care and harm, Nok managed to establish a home for her family that, while it has not always been a safe place for her, still allows for some degree of recovery and nurturance.

The Struggles and Perseverance of Phem and Yi

Phem was quite sure that the negligence of birth attendants had resulted in her son being a *luk phikan* (disabled child). Phem and Yi were the couple introduced briefly in chapter 2. For this young couple, aged twenty-two and twenty-four at that time, raising their first son became the biggest challenge of their lives. Phem had come to Thailand with her grandmother when she was fifteen years old to work as a domestic worker. During the first few years, she made good money. She told me proudly, "I once sent my mom more than 10,000 baht (around USD 300). In Burma, it was quite a sum of money. I really worked hard, working as a housekeeper during the day and cleaning buildings at night." But she became gravely ill and could not get proper treatment from the hospitals in Chiang Mai. "I later knew that I got tuberculosis, but they didn't tell me at that time." In the end, she decided to return to Myanmar. For her weakened body, a seven-day bus ride was almost unbearable. Fortunately, she made it home alive, and her mother took her to a hospital in Yangon. She eventually recovered after spending a sizable amount of money on hospital fees. She felt the guilt of spending all of her mother's savings and decided to go back to her job in Thailand. Soon after, Phem met Yi at work, and they married. When I visited with Yi and Phem's cousins, Yi told me that when he first met Phem, she was very pretty and many young men were interested in her. "Living through hardship, Phem is not like she was before. See, where is her beauty now?" "No, Phem is still beautiful," I replied, and we laughed together. It was quite true that the young couple had gone through many ordeals together after Kohn's birth.

"The hospital treated us badly because we are Shan," said Phem. When I visited Phem's new place near Yi's mother's shack, Phem had many things to say about her childbirth. Phem was pregnant the year she married: "I knew that it was not a good time to have a child. We hadn't saved much money yet. But Yi said that aborting a child is a sin. So we decided to keep the baby." Phem recounted her first childbirth experience: "When I went to antenatal care, the nurses all looked angry. I told them I had tuberculosis before, and I was worried that I couldn't give birth by myself. But they said that I would be fine." Phem remembered that when she entered the labor room one early Sunday morning, there were no doctors, only nurses. This was a district hospital in Chiang Mai that was similar in size to Ban Phaet Hospital.

Phem continued to explain her terrifying labor experience.

> The nurses in the labor room were bad mannered. When I lost all my strength, they scolded me for not pushing harder. I asked them to send me to the big hospital, but they said that if they did, I would die on the way. They tried to get the baby out, but I heard that the machine didn't work. Then, one nurse said that either I or my child would die. I was already so exhausted. When my baby came out, his body was greenish. And he didn't cry. I hit his bottom, but he didn't cry. The nurse said that the baby would die soon. Then I just fell asleep. I heard from Yi later that he was told that the baby's body had already turned green. The nurse then asked Yi whether he wanted to save the baby. He cried to them to do everything for the baby. The nurses treated us badly. After they had sent the baby to Ban Phaet Hospital, they even didn't tell Yi where the baby was.

According to Kohn's medical records, the medical staff had tried vacuum extraction, but the result was unsuccessful. Kohn had suffered severe birth asphyxia that eventually led to brain damage. After Yi's begging, the baby was resuscitated and sent to the neonatal intensive care unit at Ban Phaet Hospital. "If they had sent me to the big hospital right away to do surgery, it never would have been like this." Phem firmly believes that an emergency caesarean section would have prevented this unfortunate result, but she was never given this chance. While staying in the Ban Phaet Hospital NICU for a month, she also learned more about how her son could have been born safely.

> Phem: The doctor in Ban Phaet Hospital said that Kohn was out of oxygen for almost an hour. If I had given birth in Ban Phaet Hospital, they

could have given him oxygen straight away. When my Shan friend gave birth, she tried to push five or six times but it didn't work. So the nurse sent her to the big hospital and her child was totally fine. In the NICU, I met another Shan woman who also had vacuum extraction, but the baby spent only a day in the ward and could then go home.

Bo: Have you ever been back to the hospital where you gave birth? I once heard a story of a Shan woman who died in that hospital during childbirth. People said that her family received some compensation money. Did anyone from that hospital apologize to you?

Phem: No, they didn't say anything to me. And I didn't want to talk to them again. My Thai neighbor said that we could sue the hospital and ask for compensation, but it was my first birth and I didn't know what I could do. So I never visited them again. Yi told me, "Forget about them. *Chang man thoe* [let it go]. He is our son and we will take care of him anyway."

Phem's rancor and frustrations were deep, but she also felt that, as a migrant, confronting the medical staff with the accusation of malpractice was not an option for her.

Since his birth Kohn has required constant medical attention. And Phem has no alternative other than to rely on the Thai public health system. Contrary to their previous hospital experience, in Ban Phaet Hospital NICU, Phem and Yi eventually had developed very close relationships with several of the medical staff. The NICU pediatricians remembered Kohn's case well and often mentioned Phem as an exemplary mother who tries to do her best to take care of her sick child. The medical staff's close attention to Kohn not only originated from their sympathy for his unfortunate condition but also was influenced by his parents' dedication. Kohn was eventually weaned off ventilation support, but he was still severely underweight and susceptible to several infections and pulmonary diseases. Monthly follow-ups were needed with the pediatrician in the NICU in addition to extra eye tests and cranial ultrasounds; vaccinations; physical therapy; and treatments for skin rashes, fevers, pneumonia, and feeding problems. Phem and Yi took Kohn to the hospital on every required occasion despite living far from the hospital. On many occasions Yi's old motorbike carrying the whole family had shuttled across the highway overpass to come to the hospital.

To respond to Kohn's unstable condition and most of all to keep close contact with the hospital, Phem and Yi had to make money and find time.

While Yi drifted from one construction site to another to find work for a higher wage, Phem stayed close to her mother-in-law so that she could also go to work. While Yi's mother took care of Kohn, Phem worked twelve-hour days in a small baking factory where she earned 140 baht (USD 4) per day. Her wage was much lower than other workers as she had to go back home from time to time to check on Kohn. As an experienced construction worker, Yi earned a wage that was a bit higher than average, 270 to 300 baht per day. There was a time when I saw Phem and Yi three times in a week at the hospital, which meant that they had lost three days' wages that week. Yi once told me that the doctor's admission order was the scariest thing that could happen to him at that time, not only due to his concern for Kohn's health but also because it ate up their time and money. Whenever Kohn was hospitalized, Phem had to quit her job to take care of him, and Yi's sole income was not enough to cover the hospital bills and everyday expenses. One day I met Yi dozing on a bench in the hospital garden. What he first said to me, shaking his head to wake himself up, was "So tired."

Phem and Yi had the option of going to a district hospital nearer to where they lived, but instead they faithfully returned to Ban Phaet Hospital. Their relationship with the hospital staff was not a conventional patron-client one; rather, it was quite clear that they had developed a relationship of personal trust with the hospital and received more help than most other Shan patients. For instance, the pediatrician ordered a special fortified infant formula for Kohn that was not available in the district hospital dispensary. This kind of support would not have been given had Phem not proactively solicited it. When the opportunity arose, Phem gave a detailed account of Kohn's feeding problem and effectively caught the pediatrician's attention. When buying the special baby formula became unaffordable for Phem, the senior nurse in Ban Phaet Hospital introduced her to a Japanese charity. The arrangement was that Phem joined the charity's monthly meeting at the hospital, and the charity would pay for the baby formula and hand over 200 baht (USD 6) for the transportation costs. It was not enough to compensate for the couple's daily wage, but Phem insisted on going to every meeting to fulfill the conditions of the charity.

The social ties that Phem had developed with the hospital were not purely based on economic interests: they related to shared aspirations regarding Kohn's development. Numerous follow-up appointments with the doctor and the recommendation of physiotherapy were not regarded as burdensome requests. Instead they were appreciated as they proved the hospital staff's concern for Kohn's growth. In a similar way, a female physiotherapist around the same age as Phem also became attentive to Kohn's condition. One day when Phem came to the physiotherapy clinic, she was very upset: she told us that Yi's sister had insinuated that it would be better to drop Kohn off at the hospital door. At that time, Yi's mother was taking care of both Kohn and Yi's sister's newly born son, and Yi's sister wanted her mother to focus only on her own child. When Phem told the story, the young physiotherapist listened to her words and gave a nod of empathy while stretching Kohn's back on a gym ball. These two women, who had been working together for several months to enable Kohn to hold a small toy in his tiny hands, shared a special bond that Phem's other friends and even kin did not have with the young boy.

The birth of another grandson, who was born six months after Kohn, inevitably led to the drawing of vivid contrasts between the different pace of growth and development of the two children. While Yi's sister's six-month-old son had started to make eye contact with other people and to crawl around, one-year-old Kohn still could not cry out loud (instead he only made a groaning sound). Yet this contrast was not spoken of with disappointment. When I sat with Kohn's mother and grandmother, they rather acknowledged how he was growing: since Kohn had been on new medication, his hands and feet had become less stiff, and the number of seizures had decreased; Kohn started to make simple "e," "u," and "a" sounds; and when his grandmother called his name, he looked at her. When Phem's relatives and neighbors mentioned Kohn's doomed future, she did not refute them directly but held on to what the pediatrician had said about Kohn. "His brain has become very slow. It will take a long time, but he can help himself when he grows up," was the mother's answer to them.

Finding Strength and Opportunity

Phem's strength was in her tenacity in maintaining relations of trust instead of being consumed by rancor. Although she did not stop condemning the discriminatory practices of the Thai public health system, at the same time she actively cooperated with hospital staff to secure the care required for her child. She could not fight back against the hospital that she held responsible for her son's permanent brain injury, but she did summon the strength to negotiate with the staff at the Ban Phaet Hospital. It was clear to Phem and Yi that Thai public hospitals were not trustworthy places, yet it was equally true that they required professional help to raise their child. Phem and Yi made determined efforts to cultivate reliable connections with the hospital staff, and these hard-earned relationships have helped secure necessary medical attention and treatment for Kohn. While there were several moments when pressure from family and kin to triage care caused them to have doubts about their son's future, the support received from an extended network of caregivers sufficed to keep them hopeful about his prospects for growth.

As Kohn grew up, many things happened to his family. In May 2013, I heard from Phem that Yi's mother had died of kidney disease. Yi was his mother's dearest son. She once told me, "Yi was the only one ordained for me. When his older brothers had to take care of their own family, Yi was the one who looked after me and his younger siblings." After her untimely death, Phem and Yi finally moved to a remote hill area to start contract farming. Yi had come up with this plan a year before, but at that time they could not make a decision because they did not want to live so far away from the hospital. Contract farming was Yi's new plan for escaping from the endless wheel of wage labor that he had started at the age of fourteen. "It's not like working for others. I can have my own work." Yi's new dream was to start a small flower plantation. A relatively wealthy Hmong man in his thirties, who owned a large plot of land as a Thai citizen, became Yi's boss and *phoh liang* (patron). He provided land, fertilizer, seedlings, and all other resources, and Yi sold his harvest of chrysanthemums exclusively to his boss for a fixed price.

After they moved to their new place, I could not meet them as often as before. But Phem still went down to Ban Phaet Hospital regularly, and one day she invited me to see their new flower farm. I planned to rent a car to visit them, but Yi assured me that he could pick me up from the hospital. Soon after I realized that this trip was planned not only for me. Phem's mother and stepfather had arrived in Chiang Mai for the first time, and Yi had borrowed an old pickup truck from his new boss for this family reunion.

After many years of separation, it was the very first time that Phem's mother had met her son-in-law and first grandchild. Phem's mother, who was in her late fifties, looked very tired after the long trip and was very much concerned about her grandson. She looked at him for a while and told me that she had not expected that he would be like this. On the way to the farm, we all stopped at a small market, and Phem bought an electronic pan, a bottle of cooking oil, and a bag of MSG powder for her mother's new hearth. A small, dark shack next to the irrigated slope was Phem and Yi's new home. That night Phem's cousins gathered around us to welcome Phem's mother and stepfather, and we stayed up late drinking. Phem's mother asked me when Kohn would walk, and I answered just as Phem usually did to other people, "The doctor said that he would get better." During the night, the endless sound of water from the irrigation system flowing down the slope sounded like rain.

Soon Yi developed an idea that he would rent a larger plot, so that Phem's parents could also join the flower farming venture. Phem's parents eventually became "illegal" migrants in Thailand, but with their help, Yi could produce more crops. Yi was excited about his new work: "As soon as we harvest and sell the flowers, I can have a good chunk of money. We could never save this much money working at the construction site." However, after three harvests, Yi and Phem eventually returned to construction work. Phem had once had tuberculosis, and her lungs seemed unable to bear the pesticides any longer. "My mother felt such pity for me. She begged me to go down to the city," Phem explained to me. At this time, Phem's mother and stepfather continued flower farming on the hill while Phem and Yi rejoined Yi's distant cousins.

The couple's return to the city was not a sign of failure. With their savings they bought an old truck by three yearly installments, although they did not have a driver's license. Having their own car meant that they could take Kohn with them to work. "I felt bad that I couldn't be with him when I had to work in the field all day. Now we can let Kohn stay in the car during work, and I can check on him from time to time," Phem cheerfully told me. Moreover, having the truck put Yi in a better position at work as he transported people from the camp to the worksite and started to take charge in organizing other workers. One day, Yi organized his own crew as one of the few skilled migrant workers at the site.[12] The first fruit of this venture, the old truck, would not only contribute to Yi's construction career; it also afforded more care and attention to Kohn.

Vulnerability and Resistance

In the midst of structurally imposed vulnerabilities, these Shan women search for, gather, scavenge, consolidate, improvise, and assemble a livelihood. In this mode of living, various sources of care, such as traditional regimes of protection, biomedical treatment and pharmaceuticals, patron-client relations, kinship ties, and charities are captured, solicited, and activated. On hundreds of construction sites and agricultural farms in Chiang Mai, as formal mechanisms of social and legal protection largely remain out of reach for Shan migrants, one finds these substantive relations of care flourishing. They are not sufficient to resolve all the painful realties of displacement, poverty, and violence, but they are still instrumental in creating a livable environment.

These Shan people's homes allow us to observe not only how their aspirations for a good life are hampered by the political economy in which they are forced to live but also how they persevere despite having the odds stacked against them. Sen, Nok, and Phem and Yi faced different challenges, but they all persistently refused to remain isolated and continued to make provisional alliances. Their ability to draw out whatever small assistance is available to them to help them care for themselves and their families demonstrates how vulnerability can be coupled with resistance. Since a political language of rights or empowerment is rare in their narratives, the term "resistance" may sound irrelevant. Yet if we understand resistance not as an oppositional agency of right-bearing subjects but as a capacity to change things by making others feel and act, we find that producing and eliciting responsibility and care can also bring transformative efficaciousness.[13] In this sense, people's work of self-care, making themselves socially present, and searching for a better future is woven out of a dynamic line of resistance entwined with a thread of vulnerability.[14]

When I returned to Chiang Mai in 2016, Sen had been divorced for a year and was raising her son on her own. The baby boy was already in preschool. I stayed a night in her newly rented house, a tiny brick, unplastered shack with a sheet metal roof, catching up on each other's lives. The next morning we went to the field together to pick young *chaom* leaves under a fine but cold drizzle. When I could not hide my belated concerns about her being a single mother, Sen gently responded, "You don't have to worry about me. I'm fine. Khiaw didn't want to fight [*mai yak su*]. Weather like this, he wouldn't go to work, he didn't struggle. To me, this is nothing. I'm not afraid of being wet or getting cold. Working on the farm, making money, raising my boy, I can beat them all. I will continue to fight to make a living." This sense of strength and pride, although fraught with hardship, was what Sen had nurtured for herself.

6

Spirits and the Circuitry of Care

In September 2010, a house-blessing ceremony was held in Ban Phaet Hospital. An altar to Buddha was set up on the second floor of the main hospital building, and hospital staff and patients brought offerings of yellow robes, food, and money. The staff on duty had to remain at work, but the head nurses of each department and doctors in charge of the surrounding village health stations gathered in Ban Phaet Hospital for the ceremony. Before the chanting of prayers started, the abbot and monks from the nearby temple walked around to every corner of the hospital buildings and sprinkled holy water with words of blessing. When the monks eventually arrived at the second floor and entered the inpatient ward, patients sat up in their beds and placed their palms together, and nurses stopped what they were doing briefly and kneeled down on the floor to receive a blessing. After the purification, the abbot and monks were seated near the altar. A white string tied around the building was attached to the Buddha statue and held in the abbot's hands. Then, a senior doctor got up in front of the congregation and lit a candle. Soon the chanting and the sacred words of the monks, amplified by the microphone, filled the hospital corridor. Once a year, the hospital as a community and social body performed this ritual to make merit and be charged with auspicious power and protection.[1]

This annual ceremony acknowledges the very basic fact that the hospital accommodates the power of sacred forces. Such rituals are not unusual components of modern hospital medicine in Thailand, which is not only ruled by the principles of sterility (Katz 1981) but also occasionally requires techniques of purification and sacralization. Souls of the dead, spirits, and deities are dispersed in the hospital space as in any other place in Thailand. For example, one form of acknowledging the presence of supernatural beings and sacred forces that attend to human life is the custom of leaving coins under patients' beds for the souls of the dead who previously occupied those same beds. Other examples are the small altar in the NICU dispensary, the elaborately decorated shrine of guardian spirits in the backyard of the hospital, and the amulet under the doctor's white coat.

These practices do nothing to undermine the scientific rigor of contemporary biomedicine in Thailand. Rather, the annual merit-making ceremony and daily rituals performed within the boundaries of the hospital indicate the overlapping conceptions of life embedded in the contemporary organization of care and medicine. Providing a panoramic view of how different types of healing coexist in the urban neighborhoods in India, Veena Das notes: "Life is not simply the relations humans have with each other, but also how the inhuman—as animal, as machine, as ghost or as spirit—is, or becomes part of, the social and cultural milieu within which human beings are thrown together" (2015, 116). Therapeutic efficacy is not solely guaranteed by the biomedical model in this milieu but rather has to be distributed along the diverse relations that humans can have with nonhuman entities. In this chapter I will show how encounters with nonhuman forces open a new lifeway for people in precarious situations. I suggest that uncanny encounters do not represent a breakdown of the normal but rather conjure the possibility of accumulating power over life. By focusing on how ritual technologies are adopted to elicit appropriate mutuality between spirits and humans, I further explore the overlapping terrains of care and power.

Spirits, in contemporary Thai popular religion, appear as available but ambiguous sources of power and protection. While divine spirits and deities exist as a source of prosperity, wealth, and security, malevolent ghosts and unruly spirits also populate the local world, causing illness, misfortune, and death. As spirits embody what Durkheim famously called the "ambivalence of the sacred" (Durkheim 2001, 306), ritual technologies are actively utilized to formulate a relationship to the spirit world that benefits human beings. The proliferation of urban spirit shrines, amulet markets, and other commercialized ritual practices provides a lingering example of how spirits are invited to fulfill worldly human desires and needs.[2] Instead of approaching the commerce between human beings and spirits as a pragmatic exchange of favors, I focus on the ways in which the spirits' power over life is sensed, evoked, and transferred. As we witnessed in the cases of Sen's daily acts of asceticism and Nok's recurrent struggles in chapter 5, for afflicted people, sacred forces never guarantee a remedy but do offer uncertain opportunities. Given the skepticism among believers as to spirits' intentions and capacities, we might ask why and how human beings and spirits, these ontologically different entities, seek to exert influence over each other and collaborate despite this state of indeterminacy.

The availability of spirits and deities as a tappable source helps wire the hospital, shrines, and patients' homes into the long circuit of care. The concept of a circuit is a particularly useful metaphor here for delineating how numerous pathways through which the currents of power and life forces can flow into human bodies, local territories, and social institutions hold together. While universal health coverage composes its own circuit that allows people to access care from the state, it is still with breaks, missing parts, and loose connections to be fixed. In the following, I show how spirits' potency extends and shores up the local circuit of care from warding off danger and injury to mending hidden disruptions of everyday life. The force that drives such movement is people's work of elicitation that persuades spiritual beings to recognize and respond to human predicament and so gives them new life form as a caregiver.

Looking after the Dead and the Living

When I was doing a short survey of migrant workers' perceptions of the Thai health care system in one of the long-running Shan construction camps in Chiang Mai, Aunt Uan's story was often mentioned by concerned neighbors. Aunt Uan's long struggle with kidney disease was a case that showed how little help the Thai hospital system could provide to impoverished Shan migrants. Many of them did not know the exact name of her disease, but they remembered the painful process of her death: "In the end, her foot was swollen so big, and she barely walked," the shopkeeper who often accompanied Aunt Uan on her temple visits recalled. I had no chance to meet Aunt Uan, but her husband told me details of his wife's last three months. Both of them had worked as painters for almost ten years in Chiang Mai, and two of their sons also became construction workers.

Aunt Uan died when she turned forty. "She was still so young. She used to be healthy, not weak," Uncle Kham lamented, as he was grilling dried bean paste in front of his makeshift house in the camp. When she first began to feel sick, what Uncle Kham heard from the hospital was that her blood pressure was abnormal. After several outpatient visits, a doctor in the nearby district hospital told them that her kidneys were not functioning properly. Uncle Kham expected that she would have to undergo an operation, but it never happened. He sketched out the long battle to find a way to treat his ailing wife.

> I heard that some sort of skin, like fat, blocked the vessel connected to the kidney, so if she undertook surgery to get rid of that part, she might survive. Some people still said that she wouldn't live any longer, even if she had an operation. We had every document and health card in proper order, so the district hospital should have been able to send her to the big hospital. But they never did. The hospital must have thought that we were migrants, that we didn't have money. If we were Thai, they would allow us to pay them back later after the surgery, but we never had a chance. The doctor told me, "I know you're a migrant and don't have enough money." And he said that even Thais couldn't afford the surgery. It will cost more than one hundred thousand baht. I only had 2,500 at that time, but if he only had offered me a referral letter, I would have given her the chance to undergo surgery, no matter how much it cost.

Uncle Kham's recollection was not much different from that of the many other Thai and Shan chronic kidney failure patients I had met in Ban Phaet Hospital. People wondered why the diagnosis was changed from that of high blood pressure to kidney malfunction. It was not easy to accept that there is no recovery in kidney disease, and eventually most of them despaired at the high cost of dialysis treatment. In chapter 2, we saw the rough and painful journey of a Thai patient to get dialysis under the universal coverage plan. For migrants, the chance of getting dialysis was much lower, because the Compulsory Migrant Health Insurance Plan did not cover continuous renal replacement therapy. They were seldom given referrals to the tertiary hospitals and were therefore unable to put their names on the waiting lists. In her last three months, Aunt Uan received ambulatory dialysis only once from the provincial hospital, and then she was sent back to the district hospital. "The doctor said that she was fine to go home. Then, what could we do?" Uncle Kham told me without any rancor. As he finished roasting the last batch, we became enveloped in the salty and pleasant smell of fermented bean paste. Uncle Kham invited me and Sai, my Shan research collaborator, to come inside.

Having spent many mornings in the provisional kidney clinic at Ban Phaet Hospital and witnessing the many problems with the referral process, I expressed my dismay to Uncle Kham, to which he replied calmly, "No reason to be angry at the doctors. They are not the ones who ask us to come to see them. We are the ones who go to them to ask for help. It's our own burden, not theirs." Although Uncle Kham was still grieving the fact that his wife never had a chance for proper treatment, he was quite firm about his limited expectations of the hospital. When I asked about the quality of care given to her, he continued: "I don't want to say that the hospital was bad. Whenever we went to the hospital, they helped us. But they didn't give us the chance to undergo surgery." I was puzzled by this mixed response of grief and resignation. Later, he continued to tell us about Aunt Uan's severe pain, which prevented her from eating the food she craved and fulfilling her wish to return home before she died.

Uncle Kham was also the person who introduced me to Jao Phoh (an honorific title meaning "Lord Father") Phusohphai, a medium of Shan guardian spirits. After Aunt Uan died, his first son started to hear strange noises in their house: a rattling sound, the clinking of a spoon, and footsteps. His twenty-year-old son visited the Lord Father Phusohphai and asked for help. The spirit medium performed a ceremony to cut the attachment between the deceased mother and the son, and the sounds were gone. When Uncle Kham also went to see the spirit medium, the medium told him that his wife was staying with old ladies in white clothes. According to the medium, it meant that Aunt Uan was in *mueang phi*, a heaven for sacred beings, staying with nuns.[3] Then the medium asked them to set up a small altar in Uncle Kham's house to allow Aunt Uan to acknowledge her death and help the family stay well. The medium prepared several ritual ornaments for Uncle Kham's family and asked the family to keep this altar for at least two years. Uncle Kham's young son spent 7,000 baht in the preparations for the altar. At that time, he worked six days a week and made around 4,000 baht per month.

In their shabby makeshift shack, the bamboo floor was the only bed for both father and son. The thin torn mattress, mosquito net, burlap sacks full of clothes, electric fan, and most of their possessions were cluttered on this floor. There were two altars at the side of the room: the altar to Buddha high up on the wall, and the altar to Aunt Uan on the bottom. The white cloth on the altar and the adorned bowls separated the space from that of ordinary household items. Aunt Uan's funeral picture, which

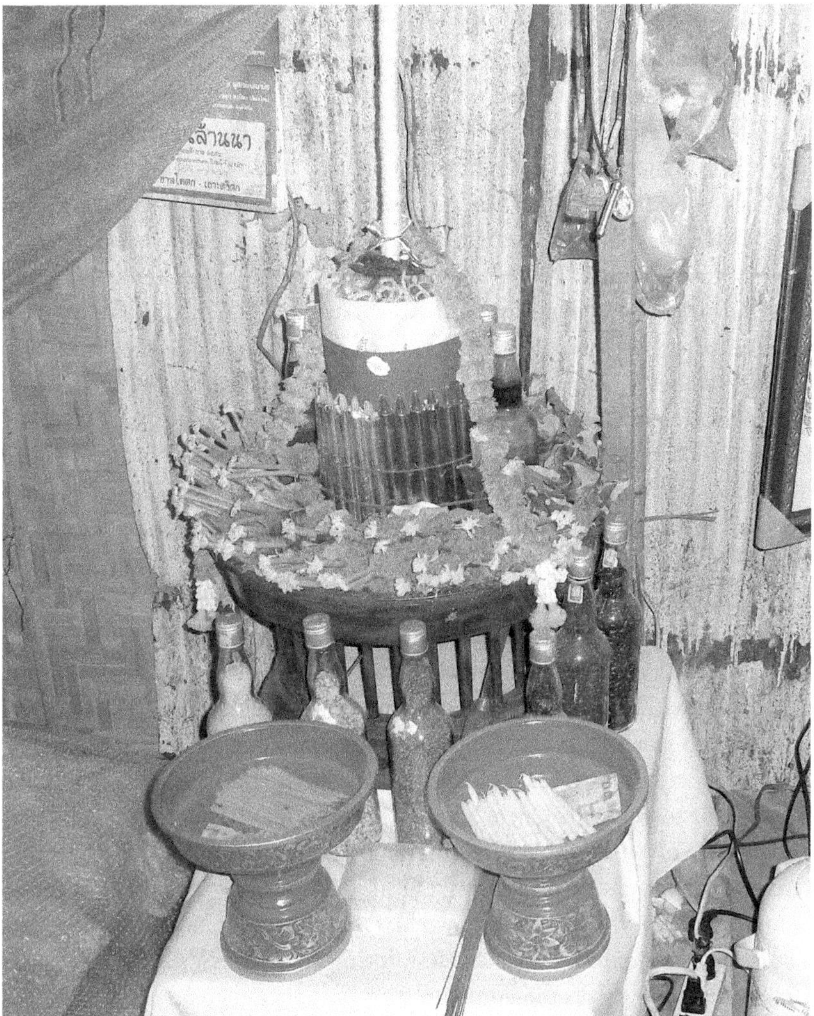

Figure 7. The altar for Aunt Uan

had been the picture on her working permit, and several amulets hung close to the altar. In this cramped space, these auspicious objects were just adjacent to the crude wooden bench for kitchen utensils. Both the living and the dead needed these materials to reside in and traverse this world.

In this family's experience, the efficacy of the spirit had to do with mending family relationships after death rather than healing the sick body. Even when Aunt Uan's health had seriously deteriorated and the hospital was not offering any effective treatment, Uncle Kham did not seek help from any spirit mediums. He thought that spiritual healing was unnecessary for a kidney patient. But when his son noticed the odd events occurring after her death, Uncle Kham was willing to follow the medium's advice. Only when the relationship between the dead and the living seemed to be unsettled did they see the necessity for spiritual care. The medium made sure that Aunt Uan had accepted her death and had taken the journey from this world to another, even though her last wish to go back to her hometown before her death had never been fulfilled. The medium's ritual intervention eventually allowed the family to continue to care for Aunt Uan after her death. By setting up the altar, they were able to reconfirm the threshold between the dead and the living, not to forget about the dead but to incorporate space for their spirits in the home.

In Uncle Kham's accounts, spirit medium–devotee relationships clearly differ from doctor-patient relationships. When Uncle Kham accepted the limits of the doctor's responsibility to care for Aunt Uan, his story was not just about structural exclusion from the public health care system based on citizenship status. It was also about the basic limits of sociality between the doctor and the patient. The hospital's failure to save Aunt Uan's life was a matter of sorrow, but Uncle Kham did not fault the doctor for a lack of personal involvement in her treatment. The spirit medium provided a different sort of attention and caring efficacy: as a mediator who could access sacred forces and supernatural powers, the medium opened up a different sphere of accountability for human suffering and pain. What kinds of sociality and mutuality do these human–spirit alliances evoke? To answer this question, I turn to the shrines of the spirit mediums.

Migrating Spirits: A Conceptualization of Sovereignty

When I visited Jao Phoh Phusohphai, he could not remember Uncle Kham or Uncle Kham's son. Contrary to my expectation of meeting with an old

Shan man, the Lord Father was a young man, living in a freshly built two-story house on the outskirts of the city. The medium was busy with a continuing stream of people who came to see him, but he graciously welcomed me and Sai and allowed us to stay. As the spirit already had descended into the medium's body, he spoke like an old man in a mixture of Northern Thai and Shan, and called me a little girl. To me, his outfit—a white scarf around his forehead, silky shirt and dark brown *phathung*—was not much different from that of other spirit mediums, but Sai, who was born in Shan State and had recently moved to Chiang Mai, noticed that he was dressed like an old Shan man.

In the middle of the consultation with one of his clients, the medium showed us a page from a book (see figure 8) and pointed to the face of the man in the picture. He asked, "Don't you think we look similar?" It was a picture of a Shan prince in a history of Shan kingdoms. I asked him the meaning of his name, but he pointed to the picture again instead of giving me an answer. In the late afternoon, when the spirit had left his body, Chom, the medium, told us more details about himself and the spirit. Chom was a thirty-eight-year-old who was born in Chiang Mai; he was the *makhi* (human medium) of the guardian spirit of Chiang Tung in Shan State. The link between the medium and the spirit was that Chom had been a prince in Chiang Tung in his previous life, and in this life the spirit found him as his medium to make merit with. Like many other spirit mediums, Chom had experienced traumatic and strange events in his life. At age eleven, he jumped from the top of a tree to kill himself, and after this incident he realized that he had to accept the spirit. He prepared his initiation ritual by himself at this young age without any help from other senior mediums. Chom has been a spirit medium ever since, but that has not prevented him from studying and working just like ordinary people. After receiving a bachelor's degree, he studied in Australia and worked in a leading bank in Bangkok as a customer service trainer. Then, five years ago, the spirit asked him to devote more time to helping other people as a spirit medium. He quit his job and returned to Chiang Mai.

That afternoon, I sat in the room and observed a series of rituals that the medium had organized for his Shan devotees. Shan people flocked to his neatly adorned shrine with a wide range of concerns. A young boy had had a fever for several days; a couple was wary about having recently aborted a child; a sick man from a remote village in Maehongson had come to consult about his deteriorating health and about his wife, who was once afflicted

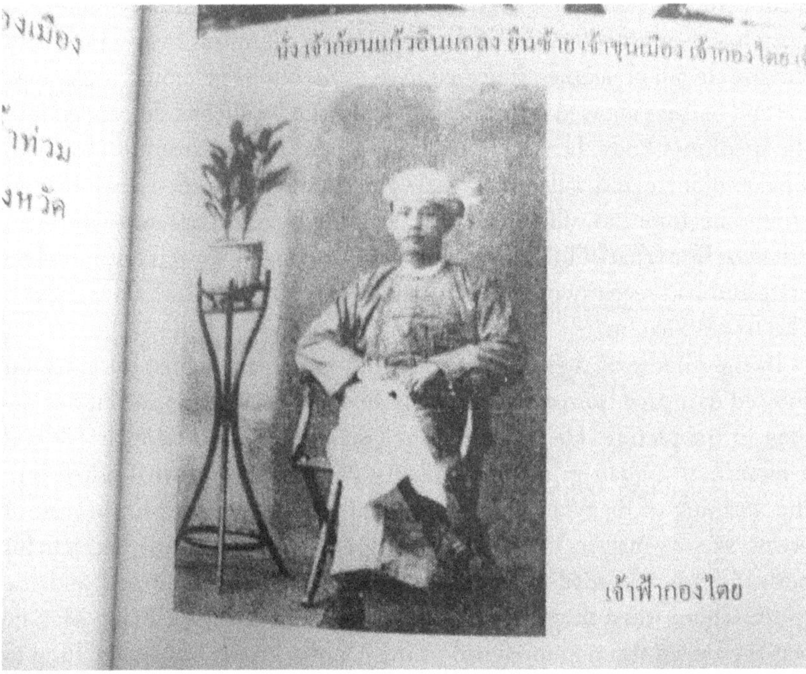

Figure 8. A picture of a Shan prince found by Jao Phoh Phusohphai in a history of Shan kingdoms

by *phi tai hong*, a wandering ghost. As remedies, depending on the type of problem, the medium offered soul-calling ceremonies, lengthy chants and bathing, life extension rituals (*sueb chata*), and protective amulets.

~

For me the most interesting aspect of this shrine was how this spirit from Shan State became a source of care and protection in Thailand. Here my concern is not with identifying fundamental cultural differences between northern Thai and Shan spirit cults. In the spiritually rich landscape of Chiang Mai, a huge number of mediums have access to a multitude of spirits from various cultural traditions.[4] Within this diverse and fertile field of cultural convergence, this shrine shows how multiple cultural markers and attributes are imaginatively recombined.[5] The sacred authority of the Shan prince in Thailand, then, is not exclusively attributable to Shan tradition, but encapsulates an ontology of power that spirits embody.

The Shan spirit's descent to contemporary Thailand is based on two elementary dynamics of human-spirit alliances. First, the activity of spirit mediums or spirit experts, *song jao* (mediating or launching the spirit), is based on the spirits' desire to be involved in human affairs.[6] Second, migration, traveling and moving from time to time and place to place, is in the basic mode of spirits. Just as people leave their original places and cross borders, spirits too have their own original territory and travel beyond it.[7] Through their movements of crossing and descending, like Doctors Without Borders, the spirits in this humanitarian convocation undertake their own journeys to alleviate human suffering. A *khon mueang* (northern Thai) medium once explained to me, "All of those spirits, of course they know each other. In their world, there is no division between Thai people and *Tai Yai* [Shan]. We all are the same humans. And these spirits all want to help humans."

These common motifs of benevolence and boundary crossing are crucial in understanding the ontology of power embedded in the relations between spirits and humans. When the medium, a reincarnation of the prince of the old Shan city, calls the deity possessing him *jao*, "Lord," I suspect that we are witnessing a metaphor for micro-sovereignty in practice. As Tambiah briefly notes, ritual enactments to access the potency of spirits have a resemblance to "the benevolent acts of the universal king toward his subjects" and contain "a rich and potent Buddhist religio-political analogy" (Tambiah 1985, 117).[8] Rereading Paul Mus's classic study of Southeast Asian religions, John Holt also summarizes the notion of power found within the Lao spirit cult as "a power that accounts for the dynamism of life associated with that locality" (Holt 2009, 24). In this rendering of spirit cults, *jao*, the lord or the deity, may refer to a concrete form of force and potentiality that has a specific reference to the local geography and historical imagination. To manifest their power, spirits and deities always require wiring in a specific territory and human life.[9]

Although Holt does not directly adopt the notion of sovereignty, I suspect that his conceptualization has deep resonance with the anthropological discussions that broadly define sovereignty as emergent forms of power over life within a delimited territory (Hansen and Stepputat 2006; Humphrey 2004). Anthropologist Bhrigupati Singh (2012, 2015) outlines the concept of "deified sovereignty" using the ethnographic example of Thakur Baba, a minor deity in central India. Focusing on the deity's potentialities of violence and welfare, he resists settling on the concept of sovereignty as "a near-totalizing force over an abyss of bare life" (2015, 43). For him, sovereignty is more about potential tendencies of power that are expressed by interactions between different forms of life. Spiritual beings have "varying relations of force and contract" (2015, 55) with humans, and based on the changing relationships between them, either life-denying or life-giving influence can be exerted.

Spirits, in this context, teach us much about the conjunctive mode of power. Their sovereign power over life and death becomes operational only when they are drawn into relations with humans. Spirits' power over life is therefore precarious in the sense that they are "in the condition of being vulnerable to others" (Tsing 2015, 20). Spirits are sovereign entities exerting influence on the living and the dead, but they are not self-sufficient: without humans, there can be no transmission and manifestation of their power. Mediums like Jao Phoh Phusohphai play a crucial role in creating and interpreting the interplay of ontologically different beings, but the outcome of their encounter is indeterminate. Healing rituals potentialize spirits' capacity for care but do not effect a promise of cure. The remaining question is what is at stake in getting involved with this kind of indeterminacy. This is not just a question about what coerces people to depend on this seemingly unreliable form of care but about how people appropriate spirits' potentiality to make their way in this dangerous world. Now I turn to a Shan and Thai couple's house in which migratory spirits are judiciously invited to dwell.

An Uncanny Abundance of Care: Protective Spirits in the Home

Noi, a thirty-seven-year-old Shan woman, an HIV-positive person and mother of three children, was the one who gave me a grounding in the confluence of caring modalities. Noi was a model patient at the Ban Phaet Hospital ARV clinic, but that was not the whole story. There was another source of care that she had relied on. In the nurse's record, Noi's CD4 counts had been in the appropriate range, but that did not mean that Noi had always been healthy. As Noi recalled, her passage through illness had been bumpy and rough. "I was so sick, I couldn't work at all. Bad headaches continued and I had no strength to work. I also felt so nervous when I went to places where there were many people. I felt terrified and uncomfortable so I went to the market only early in the day when people were not yet there. I told these things to the nurses, but they said that I was fine. I had no fever, and my blood pressure and CD4 were all fine." She told me how she had experienced pain and disturbances that were not redressed by the continuous antiretroviral treatment. Noi was well aware of how antiretroviral drugs worked and reported that she had not suffered any serious side effects from the drugs.

Two years ago, Noi and her forty-three-year-old husband, Wang, became disciples (*luksit*) of a village spirit medium. It was during a time when their health and family situation had seriously deteriorated. While Noi was not well enough to work, Wang also had to quit his job because of a back injury. The couple, a Shan migrant wife and husband from Isan (the northeastern region of Thailand), had struggled for a long time to settle down in Chiang Mai. On my first visit to their house, I had heard the long story of the blood, sweat, and tears that it took to build their home together. "I did everything I could do to make money. It was a time when I was paid 20 baht per day," Wang often told me of his young days. By taking out small loans from neighbors and employers over many years, Wang had finally completed the construction: "We eventually sold a small TV to buy wood panels for the ceiling. Poor people like us have to fight to live every day." Wang had been a hardworking father, but since his injury, his family had struggled. Matters went from bad to even worse when their first son was involved in a fight and needed a large amount of money for an out-of-court settlement. This series of family catastrophes eventually led to more recurring debt. During this tough time, Noi and Wang decided to undertake a ritual to invite protective spirits into their house under the guidance of the local spirit medium.

"I became much better since I accepted *khan* [an offering tray or bowl]. My CD4 has gone up and I gained some weight. The *thep* [divine deities], they take care of us. They tell me when I need to take a rest and where the danger is hidden," Noi told me. We were sitting in her living room where the side wall had been turned into an altar for the spirits. The altar was decorated with gold and silver tinsel trees, paper flowers, vases of flowers, candles, packets of joss sticks, silver bowls and swords, and assorted flower bunches. This exquisitely adorned altar took up a large amount of the modest concrete block house's living space. "Did it cost a lot?" The first thing that had come to my mind was the price of the ritual. "The big one for my husband is around 3,000 baht, and mine was less than that, but money didn't really matter." Considering Noi's family's austere budget, I knew that this was a considerable sum to them, but it turned out to be necessary. Eventually Wang accepted two *khan*, two sets of special ornaments for spirit worship from the village spirit medium, and then Noi also obtained one.

Rap khan, or *hap khan* in Northern Thai, refers to the practice of serving as a host of an offering being made to spirits and deities as a way of paying respects and asking for protection.[10] This is a kind of religious service provided by spirit mediums as a way to solve disciples' worldly problems such as bad luck and ill health. While this practice is often initiated at the suggestion of a spirit medium, Wang told me that he had a hunch that there were spirits who wanted to be around him.[11] "I always knew that I needed to do this. But I've rejected it. I kept saying no, no, no to the spirits. But now I cannot say no anymore," Wang recounted. Noi's *khan* was for guardian spirits from her hometown in Shan State, and Wang's *khan* was for warrior spirits originally from Chiang Dao. A multitude of spirits from different places was convened in this small, one-bedroom house.

The care and protection they received from the spirits did not negate the efficacy of biomedical care. Wang's back injury served as a trigger that made him surrender to the inevitability of being a devotee of spirit worship, but Wang continued to take medication and receive physiotherapy to alleviate his back pain after the surgery. Noi also believed that the protective spirits eventually helped her regain her health, yet this endorsement did not mean that she discredited the importance of the continuous care and treatment she had received from the hospital. Rather, Noi acknowledged the limits of care from the protective spirits as well. "AIDS and cancer are not something that the spirits can help with. It's already attached to my body, so it's impossible to get rid of it," Noi said to me, explaining why she had to continue taking antiretroviral medicine. Although Noi was convinced of the efficacy of antiretroviral treatment and the protective spirits in their own right, she asked me not to talk about her devotion to spirit worship to the nurses in Ban Phaet Hospital. She told me, "I don't want to make the nurses and doctors feel affronted. If they don't believe in this kind of thing, there is no need to let them know about this. These are just two different kinds of things. The hospital can help us and the spirits also can. And we can use both of them."

Since Wang and Noi became serious devotees of the spirit cult, they started to follow many ascetic principles in their daily lives. Wang and Noi emphasized the importance of following the five precepts, and Wang even

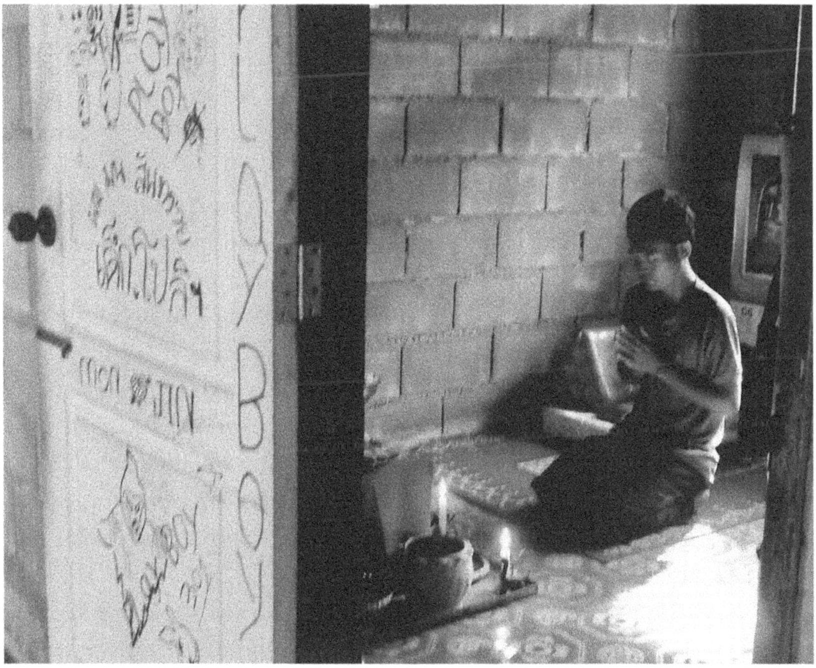

Figure 9. Wang praying at his own shrine before leaving for work. Before it was turned into a shrine, this room belonged to his teenage son.

started to add more precepts.[12] Adhering to strict dietary regimes, Wang and Noi stopped eating any meat on the Buddhist days (*wan sin*). They also stopped eating buffalo meat and killing any animals or insects. Every Buddhist day, Noi and Wang went to the temple and took a bath with *sompoi* water to wash off bad things attached to their bodies. The couple also observed sexual abstinence. Moreover, Wang studied ancient Lanna scripts and religious books by himself. He joined every afternoon sermon and chanting session in the village temple during Buddhist Lent, and Noi also joined Wang in meditation and on temple visits.[13] Compared to other devotees I had met who had also accepted *khan*, Wang and Noi maintained very intensive practices. They explained to me that each spirit had different demands of their devotees.

Accompanying their visits to the local temples and shrines, I started to suspect that Wang might want to be a professional spirit medium like others who had their own shrines and devotees. When I asked Wang whether he wished to become a spirit medium, he corrected my language:

"We don't know when the spirits will make a decision to choose us. The time hasn't come yet." In this in-between period, what Wang had pursued as a serious spirit devotee or novice medium was rather unconventional. Compared to several mediums' stories of how they were chosen regardless of their will after being "mad" or seriously sick, Wang was more driven to reorganize his life in accordance with how he felt it ought to be. He prepared trips to famous places for spirit worship and continued to join many merit-making ceremonies and prayers. He even undertook extra volunteer work such as directing traffic at the front of a busy temple in the city. These were regarded as ways of taking advantage of chances for merit making.[14] In addition, Wang obtained several amulets for his family, deliberating on which amulets would get along well with the protective spirits around him. Although Wang never explicitly told me what he aimed to achieve through spirit mediumship, it was quite clear that answering the spirits' requests and readjusting everyday behaviors had become an important part of his life and Noi's as well.

At the end of my first round of fieldwork, in early 2011, Wang showed me his own protective chants (*khatha*) that he could use for his young children. "If they have a fever, I just recite my spell and breathe into the water and make them drink it. Then they get better soon." *Khatha* is a chant of blessing that can send dangers away and bring protection and prosperity. Monks, witch doctors, and spirit mediums are regarded as having a power of blessing through their *khatha*. While some well-established spirit mediums I had met had an adorned paper or palm-leaf manuscript of the *khatha*, in Wang's shrine, there was an ordinary school notebook in which he had written several chants himself. Each page of the notebook contained a different chant for such things as making magic water for treating a stomachache; protection from robbery; invoking others' compassion; curing fever, seizure, muscle pain, or food poisoning; returning a curse from others; curing every kind of dizziness; avoiding snake attacks; dealing with wandering spirits; charming magic; and even curing insect bites. Wang wrote down each chant by hand in a mix of Pali and Northern Thai. I wanted to know more about the origin of each chant, but Wang only told me that the spirits gave these spells to him, or he learned them from somewhere. On the pages of the notebook, I could see that there were some unfinished spells written here and there, and eventually they became complete on subsequent pages.

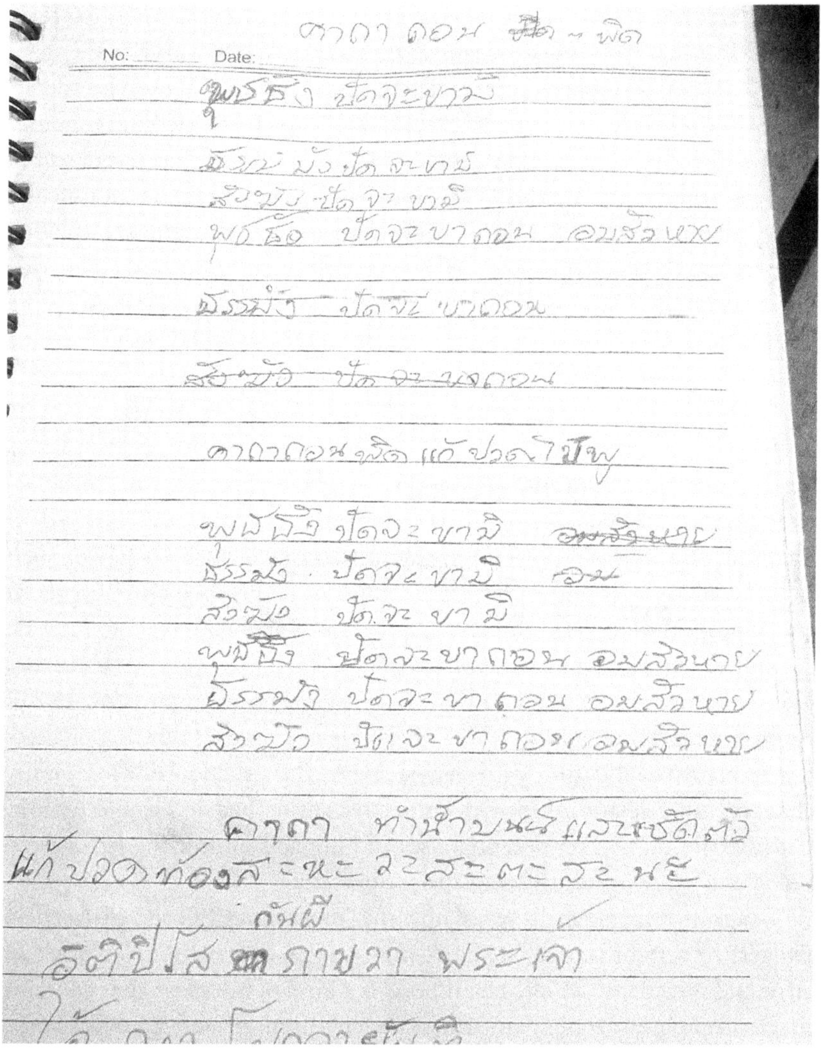

Figure 10. A page from Wang's notebook with healing chants for the following: (1) returning a curse, (2) returning a curse and using betel leaves for healing, and (3) making magic water and curing stomachaches.

Wang, who had once suffered from several afflictions, now become a healer who could administer spiritual treatment and care for his family. I wondered again whether Wang should be considered a medium, but Noi's answer was not definitive yet. She told me, "We will know when the time comes. It is just the same as when we try to choose good stuff in the market. The spirits also try to choose a good human being." Then, she added, "One time when we went to the *jao phoh*'s [village spirit medium's] house, we saw three big elephants in front of the house. All of them were so big and handsome that Wang and I saw them at the same time. I even touched the elephant with my hands. The medium told us that those elephants were for the deities. Three *ong thep* [sacred deities] all came down here riding an elephant. Only a person who has enough merit can see them." The way she told me about this mystic moment was just as blasé as if she were telling me about yesterday's visit from her neighbor.

~

Wang's and Noi's continuous attempts to adjust their way of life reflect widespread traditions in mainland Southeast Asia that are involved in accumulating spiritual power. Putting restrictions on one's behavior such as precept-keepings and other ascetic patterns of life (see also chapter 5) and relying on more powerful beings and objects are major ways to increase the power of protection (Tambiah 1984; Tannenbaum 1995). Wang and Noi's collective efforts surely fit into these religious conventions. Yet, in this run-down but other-worldly home, they were not simply following precepts but rather experimenting with new ideas. As the situation of their family changed, their relationship with protective spirits had to change with it. Creative speculation on potential uses and impacts of utilizing ritual technologies is what makes this adjustment possible.

Wang's own magic spells reveal how the "moral, magical, and ritual effectiveness of certain actions" (Mauss [1960] 1992, 460) unfold in times of crisis and insecurity. Wang's chant book is a kind of bricolage that contains magic-in-progress: some parts might be repetitions of well-known chants, and some parts might be new creations. Wang cannot explain the meaning of each verse of his own chants, just as many ordinary Thai Buddhists cannot articulate the exact meaning of Pali chanting.[15] It is not the literary meaning of each chant but Wang's bricolage and enactment of chants—making and reciting his own—that make the sacred force around him tangible and efficacious. The ritual originality embedded in his humble notebook also reveals how the techniques of the body, and eventually the techniques of caring, become creative and reflexive projects rather than prescribed rules of conduct.

However, there is no magic spell for curing HIV. This limitation of spiritual care is worth noting, not because spiritual care is spurious but because there is no universal way to deal with the complex sets of vulnerabilities that Noi and others experience. Noi's cautious attitude—asking me not to tell the nurses about her devotion to spirit worship—hints at the hegemonic position of biomedicine, but the more important aspect of this supplementary appropriation of multiple modalities of care is that both biomedicine and the potency of spirits are partial and incomplete. At a time of hardship over which they had little control, Noi and Wang did not count on a miraculous cure or rescue from either source of care. Instead they worked at cultivating and ensuring proximity to and affinity with both.

In their own way of searching for entry points into the charged circuitry of care, it is important to note that waiting and imagining appear to be an appropriate mode of elicitation for both humans and spirits. On the one hand, in Wang's and Noi's narratives of becoming devotees, the spirits' power was already present but needed to be elicited. Spirits waited to be sensed and thus invited before intervening in the family's concerns.[16] Wang and Noi, on the other hand, were also in a mode of waiting, because what the spirits' presence would effect on them had not been fully known ahead of time. They continued to observe several precepts at their own tempo, but they were still reluctant to anticipate Wang's future as a spirit medium. He once told me, "Being a medium requires a lot of self-sacrifice. I can't observe all those precepts all the time while I'm making a living. I'm a father of three children. Let's see what happens." I was unable to appreciate the meaning of these words at the time. Then I began to realize that this sense of indeterminacy and caution might have to do with a different vision of achievement than I was aware of. It was less about what the self wants to be or will be, a narrative of progress and self-creation, than it was about a method of absorption dependent upon both the destructive and aspirational potentials of life. I slowly learned about this at an unanticipated moment.

Afflictions and Aspirations

It was a quiet and cool afternoon. Noi's two small children, ages six and eight, were playing outside, and Wang had fallen asleep in the room. These days, he had returned to his previous night guard job. Noi had asked me to visit her on a Buddhist day because this year she had decided to take every Buddhist day during Lent off from work. In the morning, Noi's family went to the temple to make merit. "Is it okay to not go to work every Buddhist day? There are so many Buddhist days during the three months of Lent. I'm already tired of going to the temple in the early morning." I made these idle remarks somewhat clumsily, really wanting to ask her about how she was coping with paying the arrears in school bus fees and other bills that she had mentioned before. "It's fine. Making merit is what the spirits want us to do. We don't have to worry about money too much. Sit here." Noi insisted that I sit on the couch, not on the floor. We were sitting at each end of the old and tattered vinyl couch under the open window. The house was tranquil, waiting for the children to return.

Noi started to tell me about Wang's fruitless efforts to get her a Thai ID card. Wang had visited the village head several times to ask for help in getting formal identification documents for Noi, but he had returned home empty-handed. "The village head didn't want money. He just couldn't be bothered to get involved with any problems," Noi explained to me. "One time, a police officer came to my house. My next-door neighbor reported me to the police. It's just absurd. They had borrowed 5,000 baht from me long ago. I asked them to pay me back, at least 3,000 baht, and then they reported me to the police. I was the one who needed to call the police!" Her twenty-five years of living in Thailand and marriage with a Thai man seemed to have done nothing to help her earn Thai citizenship. Yet Noi was not as anxious about this issue as many other Shan migrants: "I don't worry about this much anymore. The police knew that I'm a mother of three children. What could they do to me? The police just went away after the village head and Wang came to our home. I was able to show my son's birth certificate to let them know that I'm his mother. Where can I go? I even don't know where I lived in Shan State."

"You came to Thailand with your mom, right?" I asked. "No, my mom sold us. My sister and me. We stayed in the big restaurant together only for five or six months. I didn't know where my mother was," Noi replied with her usual calm voice. She was twelve when she arrived in Chiang Mai. She was sold for 15,000 baht and "cried till [she] died," but her tears dried up in the end. Wang met Noi when he was only seventeen years old. Wang borrowed money from his employer and paid Noi's debt, then he brought her to his parents' house in Isan. She added, "When my sister went back to Burma some years ago, I told her that if mother asked about me, just tell her that I was dead already. Mothers should love their children, right? I don't understand her at all. But what happened is what happened. *Tham jai laew* [I've accepted it already]. If I hadn't met Wang, who knows what would have happened to me."

From her childhood story she moved to her children's. Noi found out her HIV status only after she visited the antenatal clinic for her second pregnancy: "When we heard the result, Wang told me, 'Leave it be [*chang man thoe*], everyone dies one day. You don't have to think about it too much.' But my heart was totally torn. I couldn't eat anything for several days. But the nurse in the clinic, she told me, 'You don't have to worry. Your child will be fine as long as you take ARV regularly.' She gave me such a big assurance. Then, when my daughter was born, they confirmed that she was fine after several tests. We have so much merit." Two of their children were given a therapy for the prevention of mother-to-child transmission of HIV in Ban Phaet Hospital. "If I had known earlier that I got HIV from that rape, I would have just killed myself."

Noi had told me about the terrible rape incident when we first met in the hospital waiting room. She was candid and spoke without hesitation at that time, and I was the one who could not continue the conversation in that public place. "How did it happen?" I was finally able to return to the question. "He was a Shan man who bought people from Burma and sold them in Thailand. He was a really scary man who even could bribe the police. There was no point filing a report." At that time Wang had gone to his hometown in Isan to take care of his sick mother, and Noi was staying in Chiang Mai with her first son. "I yelled. Help, help, please help me! It was a compound house in which each room adjoined. Many people lived there. A couple lived next to my room and the owner of the house was upstairs, so they must have heard me. But no one came and helped. My little son was sleeping and I was afraid that if I fought back, he might kill us." Still sitting at both ends of the sofa, we leaned toward each other, eyes brimming with tears. "How? Why did no one help?" I sighed out loud. "The neighbors must have been afraid of him. No one gave me a hand. It was so painful. Long after that, I heard that the man died of AIDS." "But you didn't talk about it to Wang at that time?" "Right, I just told Wang that I wanted to move somewhere else. Keep it as my secret. Bo, if you hurt your body, you can endure the pain, but if you hurt your heart, you cannot endure it. I didn't want him to suffer." As she said this, Noi's soft black eyes were not wet anymore.

Later, Wang woke up and invited me to go to a temple on the nearby mountain. I worried that he would later be too tired to go to work in the evening, but he wanted to take me somewhere nice. The children were excited about the short day-trip and had already taken their seats in the car. Noi also insisted that we should go to the temple to see the new Buddha statue. Following Wang's directions, I drove the car. On the way to the temple, Wang told me that the amulet that he had given me, a small wooden nail from a famous temple in Chiang Mai, would protect me during my trip back to Korea. Soon after, we arrived at the top of the mountain and went inside the temple. At the corner of the temple was Khwan Im's shrine, and Wang explained to me a bit about how to raise a *kuman thohng* (baby spirit). On the way back home, we stopped at the street vendor and had a bowl of *khanomjin* (northern Thai–style assorted noodles) together. The children also ate some sweets. Noi once told me that living a life was all about going to work, making merit, and eating together. That day, we all *yu di kin di*, stayed well and ate well.

~

I was reminded of the significance of this conversation each time I heard stories about the presence of protective power around this family. The tranquility of the afternoon and the intensity of the story made a vivid contrast—how can one be so fragile and yet strong enough to live in this world? Many parts of Noi's life story share commonalities with the stories of the Shan women we met in chapter 5. Her life experience could not be detached from the structural violence that many Shan migrant women like Sen and Nok have lived through. Moreover, during her life, family and social ties failed her as she fell victim to abuse. The lack of social and legal protections heightened her vulnerability. I had heard about the protective potency of the spirits several times, but before this conversation, I never realized the full intensity and complexity of danger, violence, and adversity that had existed in Noi's life and that of her family.

What I finally understand is that the role of protective spirits in this family's history has been to endorse and reflect possibilities for living a life with dignity. Noi's past illustrates that danger can strike one's life at any time, and the perils of life might be what makes aspiration so crucial (Kleinman 2006). Anthropologist Angela Garcia notes that an ethics of care emerges from "moments of rupture and of shared singularity" (2010, 51): although people experience incommensurate forms of pain and desperation, that does not mean that they cannot share their vulnerabilities with others. Here, I extend her meditation on incommensurability to note that not only vulnerabilities but also shared aspirations between ontologically different entities can give rise to relations of care. Experiencing numerous obstacles and traumatic incidents in their lives, what Noi and Wang have pursued is organizing the good, and spirits have become the most intimate associates who have shared and confirmed their aspirations. Spirits do matter for Noi and Wang, not because they can make life immune to danger and insecurity but because their presence allows this couple to imagine their present life suffused with potential for betterment.

In this chapter, I have illuminated how relations of care are shaped between the living and the dead, humans and spirits. By tracing illness trajectories, sites of devotion, and family histories, I have focused on the kind of power that spirits are deemed to possess and the relational fabric through which spirits come to be known and become responsible for human life. Spirits can exert a productive force that sutures a variety of human problems, not because they are an omnipotent sovereign being but because people's work of elicitation can give them a new role as a caregiver. The possibility that spirits' caregiving potential is acknowledged in everyday encounters and compelled by ritual techniques indeed gestures toward how unequal but "nonexploitative forms of togetherness" (Puig de la Bellacase 2011, 24) can be enacted within the circuit of care. Humans and spirits cannot have equal standing with respect to capability or ontological status, and the relationship between them can turn out to be harmful and dangerous. Yet when each other's presence is recognized in time and contributes to affirm the possibility of comfort, recovery, and betterment in interaction, this provisional alliance can animate both of their lives.

Conclusion

An Affirmative Politics of Care

In the end, the two men, Uncle Bun and Ek, whom I introduced in the beginning of this book, left the ward one by one. Aunt Deng's tiring days in the hospital drew to a close, when the doctor told her that Uncle Bun was likely to die soon. Without hesitation, she decided to take him home. He lingered for a few days and then passed away. Aunt Deng later told me that it was a good thing that he was taken care of by the hospital until the end and that he had then died at home comfortably. She wanted him not to feel abandoned as he was dying, and his death was eventually well accommodated by the uneven circuit of care that Aunt Deng had shored up. Meanwhile, Ek gained enough strength to pull the breathing tube in his windpipe out with his own right hand. He still could not move the left side of his body, but there was nothing much left that the ward staff could offer him since he no longer needed any oxygen support. This meant that it was time for Ek to go home. The problem was how to transport him. Phon was asked to wait a few more days in the ward, until the nurses arranged the transportation for him. She decided not to wait, because she felt *kreng jai* and did not want to burden the hospital anymore. Ek's younger brothers borrowed an old truck from the construction site where they were working and finally brought him to Phon's house. After that, when I visited her, I found that she was living in a remote, almost abandoned area. Her makeshift house was adjacent to a vast, muddy site where excavators and bulldozers were operating. After showing me the tiny room Ek was lying in, Phon told me, "It would take time. But if I help him out until he recovers enough to take care of himself, then he will live his life anyway. What else can I do?" Around three months later, I heard some good news from her. Ek had started to walk again.

The reflection I have tried to develop in this book began from the unavoidable vulnerability and dependence that these two men's feet exhibited. Aunt Deng and Phon were the ones who mainly responded to their embodied call for care. Being enmeshed within webs of responsibility, they indeed went through a hard time. The tasks of care that these women had shouldered were partly shared by the public health care system but were nonetheless deeply subjected to structural inequalities, including gendered ones. My aim in narrating the stories of people exposed to the burden of providing for the needs of others, especially in precarious circumstances, is not just about revealing the grim side of such responsibility. Rather, the effects of their care—Bun's untroubled death and Ek's recovery—although full of difficulties, attest to a transformative power that practices of care can engender. Aunt Deng and Phon would not be regarded as powerful individuals in terms of their socioeconomic standing, but they had a vital influence over the life and death of those for whom they cared. What I have sought to accomplish is to present these ordinary but powerful producers of care as well as powerful conduits through which a wider circuitry of care can be produced in the foreground.

In this book, I have illustrated the extent to which relations and practices of care are central to the lives of poor and marginalized people and to the local formation of universal health coverage in Thailand. Working with a broad definition of care, I have focused on how various lifeways intersect with and sustain each other in the local landscape of Chiang Mai. The initial puzzle that I encountered in this local context was that the poor, the hopeless, the marginal, the alien, the undocumented, and the ineligible were not simply dismissed from the realm of public health and other sources of protection. Instead, they exerted a force that entangled them in subtle but real filaments of care. As I have shown in the preceding chapters, biopolitical, interpersonal, domestic, and ritual practices of care are all instrumental in allowing people on the margins to obtain meaning and security.

A general logic of care that I have proposed calling "elicitation" throws light on this seemingly passive but in fact potent agency that brings about relations of mutuality and obligation. Let us return once more to its distinguishing features. Elicitation means that care is not simply a matter of giving and receiving but rather something in between. By reimagining care as a process and outcome of elicitation, I have illuminated what the so-called recipients of care actually do to make their needs recognizable and to prompt others to engage with them. Being a subject of care does not imply being on the fixed, receiving end of a vector of care that flows unilaterally from the powerful to the weak. Rather, I have shown how affective and material investments made by people in precarious situations open a relational field in which social others are drawn to each other. I have also illuminated how temporal and embodied modes of elicitation—waiting, maintaining, refraining, enduring, and dying—thicken one's presence and animate the effectiveness of relationality.

Elicitation indeed brings into focus the capacity for being affected by the presence of vulnerability. This capacity lies at the heart of care. Instead of approaching caregiving as a social function assigned to certain groups of workers or institutions, I have focused on the intersubjective encounters and processes through which one's caregiving potential is compelled, brought into play, and sustained. The hospital, nurses, doctors, mothers, fathers, sisters and brothers, children, and spirits appearing in this book become the responsible loci of care, only when they find themselves morally intertwined with others in need and are compelled to respond. A focus on how care is elicited in various circumstances provides a fuller understanding of caregiving not as a prescribed role or a status but as a generative ability to engage with the contingency of the self and others and to provide belonging and life-sustaining support.

In chapter 1, I have detailed how the ideal of universal access to health care was actively pursued in Ban Phaet Hospital. This community hospital's institutionalized desire to deliver care was not a mere extension of the state policy of universal health coverage but a testimony to the institution's accumulated capacity to acknowledge the local demands of care. In chapter 2, I have illuminated various affective responses that took place when the state's potential to care was elicited. Among many who have to rely on the state's provision of care, Shan migrant women's active use of the antenatal care clinic exemplifies how people in precarious situations actively adopt bureaucratic and medical technologies to make themselves as proper subjects of care and to obtain a proof of social membership (chapter 3). Creating belonging is a vital element of care even in highly medicalized settings like the neonatal intensive care unit (chapter 4). Being attuned to fragile and sick newborns' changing conditions, the medical staff provide a temporal home for them where their growth into life or death is initiated.

The repetitive practices of care are, thus, what create and sustain the pulse of life. In many Shan women's experiences of violence, terrible loss, and injustice, caring for themselves and their children appeared to be an almost impossible burden, but their care work engendered opportunities to live against all odds (chapter 5). People can also form relations of care with spirits, as nonhuman entities' power over life properly morphs into an attentive co-presence through the help of mediums or self-trained ritual technologies (chapter 6).

In all these different situations, the caring and the cared-for were mutually immersed in the receptive field of elicitation, where they became attuned to and able to be affected by each other. In conclusion, I reflect on the broader implications that elicitation has for the changing national and global landscape of universal health care and affirmative politics of life.

The Unexpected Possibilities

The fieldwork on which this book is based began in 2010. In the almost decade since then, universal health coverage in Thailand has remained in operation, yet it has also faced considerable pressure to reform its structure. The need for change arose most prominently in 2014, when the military government led by Prayut Chan-o-cha took power. The 2017 constitution drafted under the military junta narrowly recognizes the right to free health care, but only for the poor.[1] And this revision actually goes against the universality of existing systems that ensure all citizens' eligibility to access health care, regardless of their income, social status, and residency. The introduction of coinsurance and copayments has also been discussed as a possible additional reform measure to solve the financial deficits of public hospitals and to increase revenue for the universal coverage plan.[2] While the debates about cost-sharing have been renewed several times already, public opposition to the proposal has been strong as it is expected to increase the patient's financial burden.[3] For instance, the protest march organized by a wide range of civil rights groups in early 2018 called for the continuation of universal health coverage as one of the key agenda items, along with the restoration of democracy (Aekarach Sattaburuth 2018).

While at the time of writing it is still impossible to predict whether this key policy change will be pursued, it is crucial to note that recurrent debates around universal health coverage in Thailand are still not freed from the tension between the overlapping projects of paternalism and electoral populism. In chapter 2, I discussed the ways in which former prime minister Thaksin Shinawatra and the Thai monarchy appeared as givers of aid and argued that the prominence of these figures in the sphere of public health does not indicate rural people's misconceptions about tax-based state provision but instead reflects how care has been rendered as an expression of political legitimacy. The major reshapings that occurred in the two camps of Thai politics after a long stretch of military rule signal that significant change is needed in the rendering of the state's willingness and capacity for care. The Shinawatra family's political influence has been visibly suppressed since Yingluck Shinawatra was ousted from the premiership and, more importantly, the seventy-year reign of King Bhumibol Adulyadej ended with his death. Since the 2019 general elections, the long-standing political crisis in Thailand has moved on to a new phase, and amid this new political chaos, the question of political legitimacy and the politics of social provision are likely to be more entangled than ever before.[4]

Ban Phaet Hospital is one of many public hospitals that has been facing a deficit problem, yet it has also been rapidly expanding. The sixty-bed community hospital almost doubled its size in 2017 and is hiring more physician specialists in accordance with its plans to become a general hospital. Its institutional ethos of governing and caring, which I have examined in chapter 1, has become more rigorous as part of this rebuilding process. The hospital secured a seed budget for construction from the Ministry of Public Health, actively raised funds from local communities, temples, and business groups to buy new medical equipment including hemodialysis machines, and created a collaborative network among district hospitals in Chiang Mai to pool budgets at the subprovincial level. This localized scale-up of hospital infrastructure is deeply related to the social history of this institution, in which health care workers have actively reformulated the notion of universalized care in order to deal with local demand for health services. As I have shown in preceding chapters, the Ban Phaet Hospital staff have radically redefined the scope of and eligibility for public health services, enacting governmental responsibilities according to their vision of care.

Ban Phaet Hospital's growth is much needed as tertiary referral hospitals in Chiang Mai have experienced difficulties in handling an increasing patient load. The pragmatic local initiative to tackle this chronic infrastructural problem has become possible because of the hospital's long-standing relationship with local communities as well as with neighboring institutions. The social and political inventiveness that this place has embraced allows us to rethink the obligation to care not only as a moral ideal but also as a practical organizing impetus that prompts constant negotiation and collaboration within existing networks. At the national level, Ban Phaet Hospital might represent one small initiative, but it nevertheless offers a working example of what can happen when the obligation to care takes a central place in the provision of health care.

A New Distributive Politics of Care

Globally, at least 400 million people cannot obtain essential health services, and 40 percent of the world's population lacks social protection (WHO/World Bank 2015, 2017). Although universal health coverage has been promoted as one of the top priorities of the World Health Organization and the United Nations' Sustainable Development Goals (SDGs), its global achievement is a long way off (Ghebreyesus 2017). Over recent decades, even in economically advanced countries, including European welfare states, the principle of universalism has begun to be seriously undermined as public health care systems are subject to austerity measures (Karanikolos et al. 2013). An increase in what some have called "welfare chauvinism," or attempts to restrict access to health services for new arrivals and migrant groups, has been a defining aspect of Europe's response to the global refugee crisis of 2015–16 (Bradby et al. 2018).

How does this book speak to global health inequalities and how might it inform a more egalitarian and just approach for health care? In this ethnography, I have shown that public provision of health care is not an institutional machine solely directed by abstract, impersonal regulations but rather a cultivated environment embedded in local histories and cosmologies. When universal coverage is considered only as an issue of health financing, the complex moral and political ground of health care is reduced to the issue of the *coverage* itself: the creation of insurance plans based on individual coverage and the evaluation of cost-effectiveness.[5] Conversely, this book draws attention to the centrality of *care* in the everyday operation of the community hospital and reveals new dynamics of inclusion and distribution. The ways in which Ban Phaet Hospital has adopted universalistic inclusiveness as its goal and envisions such an ideal as a way to "to advance the praxis of caregiving" (Wilkinson and Kleinman 2016, 181) prove that universal coverage concerns more than just the business of funding and managing the program's budget and cost benefits. Rather, practical solidarity for continuing care is an organizing force that allows wider access to health care to materialize piece by piece in the local context.

The practical solidarity that people like Aunt Deng and Phon had to rely on, which I have conceptualized as an elicited dimension of care, reveals a rather uneasy, contingent form of distributive politics. The singularity of the lives that I encountered in Chiang Mai led me to focus on individuals whose precarious lives have made it difficult or ineffective for them to lay claim to their right to receive care. For them, eliciting care is a way of making a distributive claim to life-sustaining resources, but its outcome is often closer to dependence and submission than to individual freedom and equality. Eliciting care is not a quick, painless step. Given that elicitation is fundamentally based on one's vulnerable presence, it can be viewed as having depoliticizing effects rather than endorsing demands for rights and structural changes.

In this book, I use the concept of elicitation to expand the notion of how vulnerable people forge relations of care. My suggestion is that we expand the evidence used to examine how a politics of care proceeds under constraints. The stories in this book reveal complex dimensions of social suffering caused by structural and everyday violence, poverty, and dislocation. Yet these struggles fail to undermine individuals' tenacious claims to be subjects of care. Through elicitation, individuals can underline their concrete and changing presence and speculate as to the possibility of creating interdependence with others. Even under the shadow of inequality, a tangible sense of mutuality, companionship, and solidarity arises. And this mode of engagement fundamentally differs from the ways in which a call for action is made in humanitarian projects.[6] Rather than the abstract notion of compassion or humanity, it is people's art of presence that brings forth recognition and obligation.

Looking at the larger context of development and poverty, anthropologist James Ferguson has made a related argument about the role of presence in the notion of sharing and distribution. Addressing the extension of state social welfare programs in Southern Africa and across the Global South in which states make cash payments to their low-income citizens, he has made the crucial observation that dependence on the state and others is not a sign of degradation or a lack of freedom but rather the very foundation of politics and personhood. As growing demands for direct income payment indicate new forms of political mobilization centered on distribution itself, he suggests that the organizing principle of this emerging politics of social welfare should be "neither citizenship nor legality but something more like presence" (2015, 214). By drawing on classical anthropological accounts of demand sharing (see also Widlok 2004), he invites us to think of direct distribution as a form of rightful sharing. In foraging societies, food is commonly shared with neighbors, relatives, or anyone who happens to be present, regardless of their status or contribution. Using this model, we can think of the basic provision of care and welfare as something that has to be shared based on the mere fact of presence "here and among us" (Ferguson 2015, 215).

His argument about the heightened importance of presence with regard to envisioning more inclusive systems of distribution resonates with this book's argument that eliciting care has a progressive effect in that it creates a sense of sociality and interdependence that goes beyond the narrow conception of citizenship and entitlement. On the one hand, the relations of care that I have explored in this book entail complex politico-economic, affective, temporal, and gendered dimensions that cannot be condensed into a schematic concept of sharing or transfer. Care can be presented as both a gift and a debt, even though it is not necessarily reciprocal or repaid. In this book, I have approached care as a collaborative fashioning of life-sustaining relations that goes beyond a dyadic exchange and includes a heterogeneous set of motivations, expectations, and rules.

By accentuating presence as firm ground for solidarity and distribution, we can discern more inclusive ways in which an obligatory circuit of care takes shape. In the field of medical anthropology and in studies of science and technology, there have been wide discussions on how claims of citizenship and entitlement proliferate based on biological models of impairment and disease-based crises.[7] While this kind of collective body politic opens a space in which people's claims on the equal distribution of health resources are validated through forms of biomedical diagnosis and technical classification, its operation is closely associated with the biopolitical mode of sorting, targeting, and controlling specific populations that eventually restricts the boundary of membership and belonging. What I have explored through the concept of elicitation points out that there is a different politics at work that does not solely rely on the biological fact of being but rather rests on a relational state of being whose concrete presence demands acknowledgment.

Elicitation may not yet result in an official confirmation of an individual's right to access health care, but it has shown potential to invoke an expanded sense of our accountability for one another that goes beyond the established logic of membership and exclusion. This does not mean that people like Yi, the young Shan migrant father we met in chapters 2 and 5, did not hope for political and social rights equal to those of Thai citizens. Rather, what I want to underline is that when the liberal languages of human rights and citizenship fail to offer a substantial footing, Phem and many other Shan women are able to open a space in which their need for care can be recognized and addressed. The practical, unconditional approach to care that Ban Phaet Hospital's nurses took as their guiding principle—"Patients are already here with us, what can we do except care for them?"—shows, for instance, how the division between citizens and noncitizens, Thais and non-Thai others, the eligible and ineligible, and the deserving and undeserving can be refigured by taking into account the undeniable and unavoidable presence of others. The ways in which neonatal intensive care is organized in Ban Phaet Hospital also dramatically instantiate not the abstract value given to protecting human life itself but rather how embodied vulnerability with which everybody's life begins summons responsibility and prompts vital engagement.

The affective, moral, and political consequences of elicitation need to be detected, articulated, and amplified to make more affirmative politics of care and distribution possible. The sources and techniques of and commitments to consolidating life-sustaining relations highlighted in this book may sometimes fall short, but they have made it possible to nurture many forms of life. The power of caregiving, which we witnessed from various people's cultivated practices and sometimes from protective spirits' gestures, has to be taken as a matter of priority for social understanding and change. Obligations to care for the self and others, at times, turn out to be enabling rather than hindering, and, in that moment, the subject of care is conceived as an affirmative response to the vicissitudes of life. There is political potential embedded in the everyday achievements and failures of care. Our individual and collective capacity to be elicited can be realigned so as to produce new circuits of connections, accountabilities, and obligations.

NOTES

Introduction

1. See van der Geest (2018) for terminological complexities surrounding the English term "care" in German.

2. See also Gilligan (1982); Held (2006); Kittay and Feder (2002); Mol et al. (2010); Robinson (2011); Sevenhuijsen (1998); Tronto (1993, 2013).

3. By applying Tronto's definition to more-than-human worlds, environmentalist scholar Maria Puig de la Bellacasa (2017) points out that this generic approach is necessary to appreciate various agencies encompassed by care.

4. See Meehan and Strauss (2015); Mitchell et al. (2004). Nancy Fraser (2016) notes that the crisis of care is not a temporal condition but reflects the fundamental contradictions of capital and care under financialized neoliberalism.

5. See also Fassin (2009, 2010).

6. See, e.g., Biehl (2005); Nguyen (2010); Petryna (2002); Redfield (2005).

7. See also Fassin (2012); Ticktin (2011).

8. For an anthropological review of the multiplicity of care, see also Buch (2015) and Thelen (2015).

9. Cohen (1989)'s work is particularly important in understanding how primary health care policies were actively adopted in Thailand with paternalistic and anti-democratic interpretations. See also Lyttleton (1996).

10. See Haggard and Kaufman (2008) and Rigg (2015). For a detailed examination of the gap between state health policy and delivery in rural areas, see Whittaker (1996).

11. For example, the Rural Doctors Society had played a crucial role in generating key public policy agendas including universal health coverage. For more detailed analysis, see Harris (2017).

12. See Livingston (2012) for the uncertainty and improvisation of biomedicine within the context of universal access.

13. Singh (2013) conceptualizes this temporal dimension as the varying thresholds of life.

14. Desjarlais (2016); Langford (2009); Stasch (2009).

15. For Thai and Shan conception of the body, see Davis (1984); Eberhardt (2006); Tambiah (1970).

16. See e.g., Holt (2009).

17. See, e.g., Anderson (1972); Mulder (1979); Reynolds (2005); Taylor (2004); Walker (2012).

18. See High (2014) and Walker (2012). For a similar observation in India, see Singh (2015).

19. For more details, see Amporn Jirattikorn (2008); Arnold and Hewison (2005); Belton (2005); Farrely 2012.

20. The Shan language is part of the larger Tai linguistic family and shares many similarities with the Northern Thai language.

Chapter 1. The Government of Care

1. The rural-urban division is an important dynamic in the constitution of Thai cultural citizenship; for example, see Mills (2012).

2. The Thai Universal Health Coverage Scheme also covers accident and rehabilitation services and preventive services. Antiretroviral treatment and renal replacement therapy were excluded from its initial design, but they are subsequently included as its benefit package has been extended. For the chronology of its coverage extension, see Viroj Tangcharoensathien et al. (2018).

3. For more details, see Chutima Suraratdecha et al. (2005); Supon Limwattananon et al. (2012).

4. The complexity and multiformity of hospital spaces has been emphasized in several different studies on hospital ethnography (Long et al. 2008; Street and Coleman 2012; van der Geest and Finkler 2004; Wind 2008).

5. When the female ward is full, female patients are admitted to the male ward.

6. In 2012 the cost of Compulsory Migrant Health Insurance (CMHI) was 1,300 baht (around USD 41) per year, with a fee of 600 baht (USD 19) for a simple medical examination and a 30-baht copayment for a hospital visit. To renew their working permits, migrant workers have to make this health insurance payment every year. The CMHI covers comprehensive curative services, but it excludes several medical conditions, such as traffic accident injury and chronic renal failure, from coverage (Samrit Srithamrongsawat et al. 2009). More issues on the migrant health insurance are discussed in chapter 3.

7. The ratio of nurses and midwives per 1,000 people in Thailand has steadily increased from 1.231 to 2.295 between 2001 and 2015 (World Health Organization's

Global Health Workforce Statistics n.d.), but the nursing shortage is still one of the key problems in Thai hospitals, especially for those in rural areas. Ban Phaet Hospital is located near rapidly developing semirural areas in Chiang Mai and has less difficulty in hiring nurses than those in remote areas, yet the issues of heavy workloads and burnout are frequently mentioned, especially by young nurses. For more discussions on the nurse work environment in Thailand, see Apiradee Nantsupawat et al. (2011, 2017).

8. For extended discussions on the anthropological study of health insurance, see Dao and Mulligan (2016).

9. While there were civil society groups who advocated the most inclusive vision of the UHC that includes stateless people and migrant workers in the Thai population, in the practical implementation of the plan, only Thai citizens who have a national ID card were initially eligible for membership. For more detailed discussions on the historical struggle over this differential inclusion, see Harris (2013).

10. The paradox was that, before the introduction of the UHC, ethnic minority people who had difficulty establishing their nationality could have benefited from a targeted government health program for low income groups. To offer coverage for approximately 400,000 people registered as stateless during the delayed process of national identity verification, a new plan called Health Insurance for People with Citizenship Problems (HIS-PCP) had launched in 2010. While this policy offers a comprehensive benefit package similar to the UHC, it is reported that local health care providers tended not to fully utilize this program because of various operational challenges. For more details, see Rapeepong Suphanchaimat et al. (2016).

11. For the change of the health insurance plan for migrants, see Rapeepong Suphanchaimat et al. (2019).

12. The Universal Health Coverage Scheme in Thailand is based on a mixed system of capitation and diagnosis-related group reimbursement (Viroj Tangcharoensathien et al. 2015). The National Health Security Office allocates budgets to local providers based on the total number of beneficiaries registered with them. This means that the district hospitals' budgets largely depend on the registered population size in each locality, and district hospitals are responsible for their own financial survival (Gottret et al. 2008, 368).

13. It was not only Ban Phaet Hospital's problem, as many government hospitals especially located along the Thai–Myanmar border shared the same concern. Emergency funding of 200 million baht was given to avoid bankruptcies of affected hospitals in 2010 (Apradee Treerutkuarkul 2010), and the HIS-PCP was soon introduced to deal with this problem. While the interpretation of and adaptation to this plan seemed to be varied among public hospitals in Chiang Mai, Ban Phaet Hospital has actively utilized the HIS-PCP budget and has kept relatively stable financial conditions. For a more general report on Thai government hospitals' deficit, see Prachatai (2017).

14. The workings of the NICU are discussed in detail in chapter 4.

15. Not all nurses hired in public hospitals are public servants. The Ministry of Public Health has funded medical training to increase the numbers of doctors and nurses working in rural district health services since 1972, and under this program, many medical graduates could become public servants. But recently the employment patterns have started to change, and it has become very difficult for young nurses to obtain public service positions. Many newly graduated nurses are hired directly by hospitals, not by the Ministry of Public Health (Walaiporn Patcharanarumol et al. 2011). For the historical development of nursing as a women's career in Thailand, see Muecke and Wichit Srisuphan (1989).

16. See Foucault (2003).

17. For a similar observation of a practice-centered conception of care in Thailand, see Aulino (2016).

18. Penny van Esterik's (1996) elaboration of the Thai term *liang* is also helpful for understanding how providing care is deeply enmeshed in power relations. The verb *liang* (to nurture) denotes a broad range of actions of "caring for, tending, supporting, maintaining, and fostering" (25). It is usually used in contexts involving sharing and providing food: here, food is not only a substance of relatedness and intimacy but also "the means through which power and control are exerted" (25).

19. This combination of caring and governing might have significant implications for understanding how Thailand's modern state administration has evolved. The cremation volume of Phraya Sunthonphiphit (a key cabinet member of the royalist government after the coup of 1947, head of the Ministry of Public Health in 1946 and of the Ministry of Interior in 1947) contains an interesting article titled "the ethics of the governor," where he proposes a Buddhist ethics of care and self-discipline as a guide to modern governing. This suggests that it is worth exploring how modern conceptions of political authority have evolved in relation to notions of giving, compassion, and everyday morality. I thank Preedee Hongsaton for suggesting and translating Phraya's writing in relation to this question.

Chapter 2. Patient Waiting

1. The copayment system of universal health coverage has changed three times. Initially, 30-baht copayment for each visit or admission was enforced, but in 2006 the postcoup government terminated it. Then, by September 2012, the Yingluck government renewed the 30-baht copayment, reasoning that the increased budget would improve the quality of public medical services. In 2014, the copayment debate started again as the Thai military junta, which overthrew the Yingluck government, identified it as a target for reform.

2. See also Kuhonta (2017); Nam (2015).

3. The expansion of hospitals in the private sector received a boost from government tax incentive policy starting in the late 1980s: during Bangkok's boom

years, private hospitals mushroomed in urban areas. Between 1970 and 2000, the number of beds in private hospitals increased from 1,780 to 39,551; in 2003, 25.9 percent of the total hospital beds in Thailand belonged to the private sector (Suwit Wibulpolprasert and Paichit Pengpaibon 2003). After the 1997 economic crisis, investment in private hospitals dropped dramatically, but since the 2001 economic recovery, an influx of foreign patients and increasing domestic demand from the urban middle class have resulted in the rapid growth of the private health sector (Cha-Aim Pachanee and Suwit Wibulpolprasert 2006). In this process, it is important to note that the Thaksin government endorsed a "dual track" policy, which aims to foster a globalized private health market in parallel with the establishment of universal health coverage (Wilson 2010). This dual-track approach contains many serious problems related to the long-term sustainability of public health care and the inequitable distribution of medical and human resources between the private and public sectors. See also Chitr Sitthi-Amorn et al. (2001); Harris (2017); Supasit Pannarunothai et al. (2004); Worawan Chandoevwit (2005).

4. For more discussions on populism in Thailand, see Hewison (2017); Seo (2019).

5. A *dhammaraja* (righteous ruler) is a key concept of Theravada Buddhist kingship. This concept differs from Brahmanical ideas of the monarch, *devaraja*, or "the king of the deities," yet both concepts shape the religious and political bases for the authority of a sovereign king. See Jackson (2010) and Tambiah (1976).

6. Princess Srinagarindra, the mother of King Bhumibol Adulyadej, studied nursing and played a major role in initiating public health-related royal projects. Under her patronage, several hospital buildings and nursing schools were built, and in northern Thailand she sponsored a famous medical volunteer team that later evolved into a development project for ethnic minorities living in remote mountainous areas.

7. For more details, see Wilson (2011).

8. I was unable to find out when this incident happened or to determine the nature of the neglect. Until the end of 2005, antiretroviral treatment for HIV infection was not included in the universal health coverage benefit package because of concerns over budget feasibility, and many people living with HIV could not receive life-saving treatment. See also Padmini Srikantiah et al. (2010). For another example of ill treatment of a patient, see chapter 5.

9. See also Laidlaw (2000); Parry (1989).

10. *Kalatesa* is a Pali-Sanskrit compound from the words for time (*kala*) and space (*tesa*). Van Esterik emphasizes that "*kalatesa* is not identical to the English meaning of context . . . but to the coming together of immediate circumstances in time and space in a certain fashion" (2000, 40).

11. Based on a case study of a northern Thai family's illness experience, Cassaniti (2014) discusses several Thai idioms, including *tham jai*, that show how emotions take a key role in expressing Theravada Buddhist morality.

12. See also Eberhardt (2006); Engel and Engel (2010); Keyes (1983).

13. For the recent increase in medical litigation in Thailand, see Nanchanok Wongsamuth (2016).

14. Stonington (2012) provides an interesting example of how paying a debt of life becomes an ethical imperative in the decision-making process of end-of-life care in Thailand.

Chapter 3. Careful Inscriptions

1. On that day, a Shan spirit doctor who had also worked as a construction worker in Chiang Mai for a decade joined and organized a bathing ritual for the baby. The spiritual doctor cut the baby's hair with a razor and prepared bathing water mixed with herbs and white frangipani flowers. The baby's mother put her gold necklace and coins into water, and the spirit doctor breathed into the water and softly chanted a *khatha* (spell). After the water for the bathing ritual was prepared, the spirit doctor—followed by the eldest close family members, one by one—splashed water on the baby, wishing the baby good health and well-being. After the bathing ritual had ended, the mother and the grandmother cut the baby's fingernails and toenails and kept them to make a necklace using a strip of the mother's skirt for the purpose of protecting the baby from evil spirits and bad luck. The first month celebration for a newborn baby is often called *ap duean*: this ritual is not only for the social recognition of a newborn baby; it also signals the end of the mother's one-month postpartum practice. For changing patterns of childbirth and postpartum practices in Thailand, see Hanks (1963); Poulsen (2007); Rice and Manderson (1996); Sansnee Jirojwong (1996); Symonds (1996); Townsend and Rice (1996); and Whittaker (2000).

2. Calling and securing the souls, *su khwan* or *riak khwan*, is a common ceremony for well-being: it is also held to mark the significant occasions of one's life cycle, such as birth, pregnancy, ordination, and moving out of or into the community. For Shan notions of *khwan*, see Eberhardt (2006, 44), and for general Thai notions, see Hanks (1963) and Whittaker (2000).

3. See, e.g., Hull (2012a); Jacob (2007).

4. See also Kelly (2006); Navaro-Yashin (2007); Reeves (2013).

5. See, e.g., Braff (2013); Davis-Floyd (2004); Franklin (1997); Gammeltoft (2014); Greenhalgh and Winckler (2005); Martin (1987); Rapp (1999).

6. See, e.g., Arnold and Hewison (2005); Belton (2005); Leiter et al. (2006).

7. See Kelly (2006); Reeves (2013); Torpey (2000).

8. In mid-2014 the military government launched a stricter registration system for undocumented migrants. Under this new measure, undocumented migrants must register with the Ministry of Interior to receive a residence permit and undertake the nationality verification process, and those who fail to complete required processes are subject to deportation. The key problem at this phase was that the registration process was delayed significantly and lacked consistency. For

more details on the health implications of the changes of migration policies, see Rapeepong Suphanchaimat et al. (2019).

9. Thailand follows the jus sanguinis citizenship model (based on the parents' citizenship), and in many cases Thailand-born children who have at least one parent with long-term residency status may apply for Thai citizenship.

10. The total number of births within migrant populations from 2004 to 2006 must be much higher than 33,300. This report did not cover all provinces in Thailand and only included registered migrant workers.

11. These data are based on the analysis of the Ban Phaet Hospital antenatal clinic patient registration log from 2007 to 2010.

12. Compulsory Migrant Health Insurance (CMHI) is for documented migrant workers and provides general inpatient and outpatient services, medical referral, and medicines covered by the national drug list. At the time of my fieldwork, migrant workers had to pay 600 baht for health screening and 1,300 baht for a yearly membership. While the documented migrant workers are covered by CMHI, those who do not have a Thai citizenship but have some sorts of identification are largely uncovered or have to pay out of pocket. Prior to the establishment of universal coverage, some of them could benefit from a targeted government health program for low-income groups with their ID cards, but under the UC system people without a Thai national ID card eventually lacked access or had limited access to health services based on their residency area and card type. To offer coverage for these people, a new plan called Health Insurance for People with Citizenship Problems launched in 2010, yet to benefit from this program, people still have to get through the nationality verification process. In Ban Phaet Hospital, when uninsured people cannot afford out-of-pocket-payments, the hospital still offers antenatal and delivery care. The unpaid expenses are settled as personal debts, yet the hospital does not require repayment unless the debtors pay voluntarily.

13. Nurses advise pregnant women to come to the prenatal clinic at least four times. A routine prenatal care schedule for low-risk women in the public hospital is monthly visits for the first two trimesters (weeks 1–28), biweekly visits from week 28 to 36, and weekly visits after week 36.

14. Alice Street provides an interesting example of how patients in a Papua New Guinean hospital carefully manage their health cards to become "visible to a state that is otherwise blind to their existence and needs" (2012, 15). She emphasizes the relational capacity of such bureaucratic devices.

15. Since 2005, the Thai government has committed to providing free primary education for all children, regardless of nationality. According to a resolution of the Thai cabinet in 2005, children without documentation can access public education. Nevertheless, migrant mothers still put strong emphasis on having proper birth certification and vaccination records for school enrollment. For details of Thailand's education policy for children without citizenship, see Thithimadee Arphattanano (2012).

16. Highlanders Cards are issued to give residential status to ethnic minorities who do not have Thai citizenship. For details, see Pitch Pongsawat (2007, 176–81).

17. Two legal issues concern Shan migrant children. First, if their parents have illegally left Myanmar, the children may be ineligible for citizenship under the Myanmar Citizenship Act (Nyo Nyo 2001). Second, during their residency in Thailand, migrant families cannot travel to register their children's births to the Myanmar authorities, and without birth and household registration records it may be impossible for them to apply for an identification card in Myanmar (Yang 2007).

18. Children's right to a nationality is affirmed by several UN instruments, including Article 24 (3) of the International Covenant on Civil and Political Rights, Article 7 of the Convention on the Rights of Children, and Article 15 of the Universal Declaration of Human Rights.

19. See also Castañeda (2008); De Genova (2002); Holmes (2013); Willen (2005, 2012).

Chapter 4. Premature Life and Death

1. For a sampling of the literature in social science research on neonatal medicine, see Anspach (1987); Cadge and Catlin (2006); Frohock (1986); Lantos (2001); Mesman (2008); Seymour (2001); Weiner (2009).

2. Brinchmann and Nortvedt (2001) provide an interesting discussion of how doctors and nurses interpret premature infants' vulnerability and vitality as a key ethical appeal to care in NICUs.

3. See Carsten (1997) for kinship as a process.

4. See also Fassin (2009) for more discussions on the differential valuation of human lives within the workings of biopolitics.

5. A crucial dimension that I am unable to address in this ethnographic context is mothers' experiences, in particular of violence and suffering inflicted by anti-abortion laws in Thailand. Under the current punitive approach to abortion, poor women like Suthep's mother have no choice but to give birth to unwanted children because they cannot access safe abortion services and care. For the criminalization of abortion and its moral stigmatization in Thailand, see Whittaker (2004).

6. Based on an ethnographic study in British NICUs, Alderson and her colleagues (2005) emphasize that premature babies are not nonpersons who lack consciousness and the capacity to interact with others but rights-bearing subjects who can actively participate in and influence caring processes.

7. For an overview of Buddhist conceptions of karma, see Keyes and Daniel (1983). In the context of contemporary northern Thailand, work by Engel and Engel (2010) on personal injuries, by Pranee Liamputtong et al. (2013) on women living with HIV/AIDS, and by Cassaniti (2014) on family crisis note the centrality of karma in people's causal explanations of misfortune and illness.

8. *Ploi* is an everyday word that conveys intentions and feelings of detachment. Cassaniti (2014) offers an eloquent analysis of how this feeling of letting go is mobilized in relation to a broader Buddhist moral metaphysics.

9. See Mol (2008) for more discussions on the logic of care.

10. For more discussions on the dialectics of intimacy and separation in making relations, see Stasch (2009).

11. One of the local explanations is that the newly born baby's fontanel, the soft spot on the skull, is not closed yet, so the baby's spirit can easily go back to the world of spirit, and its body does not need to be cremated.

12. See also Eberhardt (2006); Ladwig (2012); Langford (2009).

13. Feminist philosopher Adriana Cavarero offers a related observation of the essence of nurturing. She writes: "'Mother' . . . is thus above all the name for an inclination toward the other—or, . . . , for a function that summons the requisite responsibility in the inaugural scene of a human condition in which the absolutely vulnerable—the defenseless—becomes an essential figure, first for ontology and politics, and then for ethics" (2016, 104).

14. See also Lévinas (1981, 91).

15. Anthropologist Hannah Brown (2010) shows how fear and respect, forming a particular kind of relationship based on emotional distance, become a key feature of Kenyan health care.

Chapter 5. Vulnerability and Nurturance at Home

1. For a more general introduction to the contemporary crisis of care as an innate contradiction of capitalism, see Fraser (2016).

2. Structural violence has been a central category for analyzing the historical and political-economic oppression imposed on marginalized populations, as several anthropologists working on global health inequality, poverty, and migration have shown. See also Bourgois and Schonberg (2009); Farmer (1996, 2003, 2004); Green (2009); Gupta (2012); Holmes (2013); Scheper-Hughes (1992, 2008).

3. For the wide variations and commonalities of reproductive practices in Southeast Asia, see Rice and Manderson (1996).

4. In the northern Thailand ethno-medical model, *lom* (wind/air) is an important element to keep humoral balance. For details of the Thai-Yunnan ethno-medical model, see also Irvine (1982). After giving birth, a woman's body is assumed to lose much blood and air/wind and becomes highly susceptible to disease. Several postpartum practices, including taking herbal medicines, are adopted to restore humoral balance. The local practices of pregnancy, birth, and postpartum care have been well documented around various regions in Thailand: the central region (Hanks 1963), Northern Thailand (Mougne 1975; Muecke 1979; Pranee Liamputtong 2004), and northeastern Thailand (Poulsen 1984, 2007; Whittaker 2000).

5. Mougne's (1975) and Irvine's (1982) classic ethnographies present detailed information about prohibition rules and the common complaints of wind affliction.

6. Sen did not explain all her dietary choices with direct reference to the humoral system, but she emphasized that the balance of old and new blood after childbirth is key: during childbirth, she lost all her old blood, and her body started to be filled with new blood. This new blood could be very susceptible to various foods. Based on his research on texts for ancient medicine and local belief, Irvine (1982, 115) noted that the Thai-Yuan humoral system consisted of bile, phlegm, wind, and blood. I could not collect much information about how northern Thai and Shan understandings of the humoral balance were different: most of my Shan informants emphasized the commonality between the two and sometimes actively took advice from their Thai neighbors.

7. Here Sen made an implicit link between mother's blood and breast milk.

8. When presenting Sen's experience at an academic conference, I once received a comment that describing her "smell" is rather insensitive and unethical. As smelling someone's body entails various affective connotations, what I aim to point out is that smell confirms bodily transformation in a concrete way and so helps us appreciate how the body achieves a different intensity of life. Tsing's illumination helps me think of smell as a knot of encounters: "Smell, unlike air, is a sign of the presence of another, to which we are already responding. Response always takes us somewhere new; we are not quite ourselves anymore—or at least the selves we were, but rather ourselves in encounter with another" (2015, 47).

9. For more details on acquiring power by ascetic practices, see Reynolds (2005); Tambiah (1984).

10. For the details of the home visit process of Ban Phaet Hospital, see chapter 1.

11. This is the Thai translation of the Korean-English term "Fighting!" which means "You can do it!" or "Go, team!" This expression has become widely used among young people influenced by Korean culture.

12. To be a *chang yai*, a well-skilled worker, one should know various techniques and skills involved in construction, including wiring and plumbing. This type of skilled worker would have a chance to be a foreman and a small contractor. In my research at several construction sites in Chiang Mai, it was very rare to find undocumented Shan migrant workers who had reached such middle management positions.

13. For more detailed discussions about the problem of equating agency with resistance, see Ahearn (2001). Here I do not intend to link the work of care with romantic notions of everyday resistance. Instead I am interested in recognizing the power and agency innate to the very processes of social reproduction and taking on responsibilities. Work by Laidlaw (2010) and Kean (2016) provides key insights in understanding human agency in the conceptions of responsibility, efficacy, and ethical life.

14. Butler argues that if we understand vulnerability as a "deliberate exposure to power," being vulnerable is already part of "the very meaning of political resistance as an embodied enactment" (2016, 22). My ethnographic account does not

show people's deliberate tactics for political opposition. Yet the structured and embodied vulnerabilities that encompass these people's lives and their bodily exposure allow us to appreciate that being vulnerable is not the "hallow of a power to act" (Ferrarese 2016, 157); rather, it is constitutive of the ethics of care and alternative configurations of power.

Chapter 6. Spirits and the Circuitry of Care

1. Stonington (2012) provides an apt description of how hospitals are perceived as dangerous places harboring potentially dangerous spirits.

2. For the rise of prosperity religion in contemporary Thailand, see Jackson (1999a); Wilson (2008); McDaniel (2011).

3. The conversation with Uncle Kham was mainly in the Northern Thai language, yet *mueang phi* is a Shan word. The medium seemed to confirm that Aunt Uan's spirit was with "the spirits of virtuous dead who are not yet reborn but who are 'in a good place,' that is, not hungry and wandering the earth" (Eberhardt 2006, 185–86).

4. Suriya Samutkhupt et al. (1996) suggested four main categories that are used to sort the myriad of spirits found in Thai mediumship in the 1990s: various Hindu deities, Brahma, Chinese deities, and wandering spirits were all channeled by Thai mediums (cited in Jackson [2004, 362]). Golomb (1984) gives an interesting illustration of a Buddhist curer who was also competent in accessing several different ethnic and literary sources of supernatural powers, including Muslim occult techniques and Khmer magic.

5. For example, he used black threads for rituals instead of white ones; he had no problem in addressing his devotees by their names; he did not join in any annual ceremonial dancing, unlike other Chiang Mai mediums who make a great show of organizing these. Several old *yantra* clothes covered with ancient scripts from a Shan town were also proudly presented to us, emphasizing his Shan origin.

6. The most common explanation for their desire to help is that spirits and deities are also willing to acquire religious merit for their own sakes. Jackson (2004) locates the general link between merit making and spirit mediumship within syncretic Brahmanical and Buddhist symbolism: "Immaterial beings inhabiting the Brahmaoloka heaven do not possess the physical form needed to perform good deeds on earth. These beings are incapable of acquiring the additional religious merit that would permit them to ascend to a yet higher heaven, or alternatively to attain the ultimate salvation of *nirvana*" (Jackson 2004, 363). Like human beings, even spirits inhabiting heaven need to boost their store of religious merit, and for this the spirits need a human medium. For a common local interpretation of spirit mediumship and merit making in the Chiang Mai context, see also Wijeyewardene (1981).

7. Holy High (2006, 262) shows how the spirit of the place is "itself 'extraverted' and 'travelling' rather than 'rooted'" in the context of Lao territorial spirit

cults. Discussing the effect of migration on religious resurgence in Vietnam, Philip Taylor also notes that the mobility of spirits indicates "relationships between people and places of considerable complexity, extension, and dynamism" (2004, 114). The Southeast Asia diasporas' accounts of death and kinship also vividly reveal the translocality of spirits. See Langford (2005) and Tapp (2010).

8. Wijeyewardene also pointed out that in Chiang Mai spirits are often, but not always, related to or owe allegiance to the original "lord." When people differentiate *jao phoh* (Lord Father) from *jao phi* (Lord Elder Brother) and *jao noi* (Little Lord), what is important is their different characteristics and capabilities, not their hierarchy (1981, 7). Craig Reynolds succinctly summarizes how Buddhist ideas of power can be glossed in terms of "potency, potentiality, sovereignty, and the ascetic body" (2005, 226).

9. See also Herzfeld (2016) and Morris (2000).

10. *Rap khan* literally means to receive a bowl or tray. In central Thai, the verb form "to receive" is *rap*, but in Northern Thai the "r" sound is often changed to "h." Jackson offers a detailed analysis of the symbolic meaning of *khan*: *rap khan* refers not only to the phase of accepting the symbolic bowl or tray but also to "the spirit becoming embodied by 'receiving the body' . . . of the human medium" (2004, 364–65). The *khan* has a double meaning in that it indicates the ceremonial container as well as the spirit medium's body, a human vessel that is prepared for the possessing spirits. I thank one of the editors of this series for insights on this ritual.

11. In Chiang Mai, where spirit mediumship has held a key position in popular religion and northern Thai matrilineages, it is easy to find a consultation service for home-based professional spirit mediums or small shrines of lay people who pay their respects (Hale 1979; McMorran 1984; Wijeyewardene 1981, 1986).

12. For the links between precept keeping, potency, and power in Thailand, see Reynolds (2005); Tambiah (1984); and Tannenbaum (1995).

13. The Buddhist Lenten season lasts for three months, from the full moon of the tenth month to the full moon of the first month, during which time there are thirteen holy or Buddhist days (*wan sin*). These three months are regarded as a "period of retreat and isolation from worldly affairs by the clergy, and of piety and asceticism on the part of the laity" (Davis 1984, 180).

14. Here, Wang's pursuit of merit making, which was encouraged by the spirits' requests, shows the "mutual accommodation between Buddhism and the spirit cults" (Tambiah 1970, 377). Dealing with contemporary religious repertoires in Thailand, Justin McDaniel summarizes this complementary dimension as an "ongoing and nonteleological process of creating Buddhism person by person, ghost by ghost" (2011, 230).

15. In his contemporary study of Thai Buddhism, McDaniel (2011) shows how the ritual efficacy of protective chants is widely accepted, practiced, and reinvented as a part of contemporary Thai religious life.

16. Sophie Day (2015) notes that waiting is associated with much more active connotations than the notion of queuing if we consider the Middle English sense of "waiting on" as attending, assisting, attending to, or serving without assuming a relation of subservience.

Conclusion

1. Section 51 of the 2007 constitution reads, "A person shall enjoy an equal right to receive appropriate and standard public health care." By contrast, Section 47 of the 2017 constitution deliberately omits the terms *equal*, *appropriate*, and *standard* and reads: "A person shall have the right to receive public health services provided by the State. An indigent person shall have the right to receive public health services provided by the State free of charge as provided by law."

2. For a brief report on the reform plan for introducing copayment, see Chularat Saengpassa (2018).

3. Other major opponents of the universal coverage policy are medical professionals who are associated with the private hospital sector. For more details of the medical profession's reaction to this policy, see Harris (2017, 59–62).

4. In the 2019 elections, the pro-junta party Phalang Pracharat did not win the largest number of seats, but General Prayuth Chan-Ocha was brought back as prime minister, retaining the military's grip on power. This is because the constitution, drafted by the military in 2016, ensures that the 250-seat senate is entirely appointed, and the prime minister does not need to be a sitting member of parliament. For more analysis of the 2019 election result, see Termsak Chalermpalanupap (2019).

5. For an ethnographic investigation of how a neoliberal health care reform that puts cost benefit first can bring catastrophic health outcomes for the poor, see Keshavjee (2014). For a critical response toward using universal health coverage as a neoliberal development agenda, see Abadía-Barrero and Bugbee (2019).

6. Didier Fassin notes that while humanitarian projects are fundamentally based on the discourses of compassion, such moral reason is "always directed from above to below, from the more powerful to the weaker, the more fragile, the more vulnerable—those who can generally be constituted as victims of an overwhelming fate" (2012, 4). For more anthropological discussions of the perils of humanitarian care, see Bornstein and Redfield (2010); Ticktin (2011).

7. See, e.g., Nguyen (2010); Petryna (2002); Rabinow (1992); Rose and Novas (2004).

REFERENCES

Aekarach Sattaburuth. 2018. "'We Walk' Ends with Pledge to Uphold Democracy." *Bangkok Post*, February 17.

Abadía-Barrero, César Ernesto, and Mary Bugbee. 2019. "Primary Health Care for Universal Health Coverage? Contributions for a Critical Anthropological Agenda." *Medical Anthropology* 38 (5): 427–35.

Agamben, Giorgio. 1998. *Homo Sacer: Sovereign Power and Bare Life*. Stanford: Stanford University Press.

Ahearn, Laura. 2001. "Language and Agency." *Annual Review of Anthropology* 30 (1): 109–37.

Alderson, Priscilla, Joanna Hawthorne, and Margaret Killen. 2005. "The Participation Rights of Premature Babies." *International Journal of Children's Rights* 13 (1): 31–50.

Amporn Jirattikorn. 2008. "Migration, Media Flows and the Shan Nation in Thailand." PhD diss., University of Texas at Austin.

Anderson, Benedict. 1972. "The Idea of Power in Javanese Culture." In *Culture and Politics in Indonesia*, edited by Claire Holt, 1–70. Ithaca, NY: Cornell University Press.

Anspach, Renee. 1987. "Prognostic Conflict in Life-and-Death Decisions: The Organization as an Ecology of Knowledge." *Journal of Health and Social Behavior* 28 (3): 215–31.

Apiradee Nantsupawat et al. 2011. "Impact of Nurse Work Environment and Staffing on Hospital Nurse and Quality of Care in Thailand." *Journal of Nursing Scholarship* 43 (4): 426–32.

———. 2017. "Effects of Nurse Work Environment on Job Dissatisfaction, Burnout, Intention to Leave." *International Nursing Review* 64 (1): 91–98.

Appadurai, Arjun. 2004. "The Capacity to Aspire: Culture and the Terms of Recognition." In *Culture and Public Action*, edited by Vijayendra Rao and Michael Walton, 59–84. Stanford: Stanford University Press.

Apradee Treerutkuarkul. 2010. "Cabinet OKs New Health Package." *Bangkok Post*, March 24.

Aretxaga, Begoña. 2003. "Maddening States." *Annual Review of Anthropology* 32:393–410.

Arnold, Dennis, and Kevin Hewison. 2005. "Exploitation in Global Supply Chains: Burmese Workers in Mae Sot." *Journal of Contemporary Asia* 35 (3): 319–40.

Aulino, Felicity. 2016. "Rituals of Care for the Elderly in Northern Thailand: Merit, Morality, and the Everyday of Long-Term Care." *American Ethnologist* 43 (1): 91–102.

Auyero, Javier. 2012. *Patients of the State: The Politics of Waiting in Argentina*. Durham, NC: Duke University Press.

Bamber, Scott. 1997. "The Thai Medical Profession and Political Activism." In *Political Change in Thailand: Democracy and Participation*, edited by Kevin Hewison, 233–50. New York: Routledge.

Bauman, Zygmunt. 1998. *Work, Consumerism and the New Poor*. Philadelphia: Open University Press.

Belton, Suzanne. 2005. "Borders of Fertility: Unwanted Pregnancy and Fertility Management by Burmese Women in Thailand." PhD diss., University of Melbourne.

Berchick, Edward, Emily Hood, and Jessica C. Barnett. 2018. "Current Population Reports." In *Health Insurance Coverage in the United States: 2017*. Washington, DC: US Government Printing Office.

Biehl, João. 2005. *Vita: Life in a Zone of Social Abandonment*. Berkeley: University of California Press.

Biehl, João, and Peter Locke. 2010. "Deleuze and the Anthropology of Becoming." *Current Anthropology* 51 (3): 317–51.

Bornstein, Erica, and Peter Redfield. 2010. *Forces of Compassion: Humanitarianism between Ethics and Politics*. Santa Fe: School for Advanced Research Press.

Bourdieu, Pierre. 1977. *Outline of a Theory of Practice*. Translated by Richard Nice. Cambridge: Cambridge University Press.

———. 1984. *Distinction: A Social Critique of the Judgement of Taste*. Translated by Richard Nice. Cambridge, MA: Harvard University Press.

Bourgois, Philippe, and Jeff Schonberg. 2009. *Righteous Dopefiend*. Berkeley: University of California Press.

Bradby, Hannah, Rachel Humphris, and Beatriz Padilla. 2018. "Universalism, Diversity and Norms: Gratitude, Healthcare and Welfare Chauvinism." *Critical Public Health* (Published Online Only): 1–13. https://doi.org/10.1080/09581596.2018.1522420

Braff, Lara. 2013. "Somos Muchos (We Are So Many)." *Medical Anthropology Quarterly* 27 (1): 121–38.

Brinchmann, Berit Støre, and Per Nortvedt. 2001. "Ethical Decision Making in Neonatal Units: The Normative Significance of Vitality." *Medicine, Health Care and Philosophy* 4 (2): 193–200.

Brown, Hannah. 2010. "'If We Sympathise with Them, They'll Relax': Fear/Respect and Medical Care in a Kenyan Hospital." *Medische Anthropologie* 22 (1): 125–42.

Brown, Wendy. 2004. "Finding the Man in the State." In *The Anthropology of the State: A Reader*, edited by Aradhana Sharma and Akhil Gupta, 187–210. Oxford: Blackwell.

Buch, Elana D. 2015. "Anthropology of Aging and Care." *Annual Review of Anthropology* 44 (1): 277–93.

Butler, Judith, Zeynep Gambetti, and Leticia Sabsay. 2016. *Vulnerability in Resistance*. Durham, NC: Duke University Press.

Cadge, Wendy, and Elizabeth Catlin. 2006. "Making Sense of Suffering and Death: How Health Care Providers Construct Meaning in a Neonatal Intensive Care Unit." *Journal of Religion and Health* 45 (2): 248–63.

Candea, Matei. 2010. "'I Fell in Love with Carlos the Meerkat': Engagement and Detachment in Human-Animal Relations." *American Ethnologist* 37 (2): 241–58.

Carsten, Janet. 1997. *The Heat of the Hearth: The Process of Kinship in a Malay Fishing Community*. Oxford: Oxford University Press.

Cassaniti, Julia. 2014. "Moralizing Emotion: A Breakdown in Thailand." *Anthropological Theory* 14 (3): 280–300.

Castañeda, Heide. 2008. "Paternity for Sale." *Medical Anthropology Quarterly* 22 (4): 340–59.

Cavarero, Adriana. *Inclinations: A Critique of Rectitude*. Stanford: Stanford University Press, 2016.

Cha-Aim Pachanee and Suwit Wibulpolprasert. 2006. "Incoherent Policies on Universal Coverage of Health Insurance and Promotion of International Trade in Health Services in Thailand." *Health Policy and Planning* 21 (4): 310–18.

Chitr Sitthi-Amorn, Ratana Somrongthong, and Wattana S. Janjaroen. 2001. "Economic and Health Care Restructuring: The Need for Better Governance." *International Journal of Epidemiology* 30 (4): 717–19.

Chularat Saengpassa. 2018. "People to Pay More for Medical Care under Healthcare Reform." *The Nation*, April 23.

Chutima Suraratdecha, Somying Saithanu, and Viroj Tangcharoensathien. 2005. "Is Universal Coverage a Solution for Disparities in Health Care? Findings from Three Low-Income Provinces of Thailand." *Health Policy* 73 (3): 272–84.

Cohen, Lawrence. 2004. "Operability: Surgery at the Margin of the State." In *Anthropology in the Margins of the State*, edited by Veena Das and Deborah Poole, 165–90. Santa Fe, NM: School of American Research Press.

Cohen, Paul. 1989. "The Politics of Primary Health Care in Thailand, with Special Reference to Non-Government Organizations." In *The Political Economy of Primary Health Care in Southeast Asia*, edited by Paul Cohen and John Purcal, 159–76. Canberra: Australian Development Studies Network.

Dao, Amy, and Jessica Mulligan. 2015. "Toward an Anthropology of Insurance and Health Reform." *Medical Anthropology Quarterly* 30 (1): 5–17.

Das, Veena. 2010. "Engaging the Life of the Other." In *Ordinary Ethics: Anthropology, Language, and Action*, edited by M. Lambek, 376–99. New York: Fordham University Press.

———. 2015. *Affliction: Health, Disease, Poverty*. New York: Fordham University Press.

Das, Veena, and Deborah Poole. 2004. *Anthropology in the Margins of the State*. Santa Fe, NM: School of American Research Press.

Davis, Richard. 1984. *Muang Metaphysics: A Study of Northern Thai Myth and Ritual*. Bangkok, Thailand: Pandora.

Davis-Floyd, Robbie. 2004. *Birth as an American Rite of Passage*. Berkeley: University of California Press.

Day, Sophie. 2015. "Waiting and the Architecture of Care." In *Living and Dying in the Contemporary World: A Compendium*, edited by Veena Das and Clara Han, 167–84. Berkeley: University of California Press.

De Genova, Nicholas. 2002. "Migrant 'Illegality' and Deportability in Everyday Life." *Annual Review of Anthropology* 31:419–47.

Desjarlais, Robert. 2016. *Subject to Death: Life and Loss in a Buddhist World*. Chicago: University of Chicago Press.

Drèze, Sen, and Amartya Sen. 2013. *An Uncertain Glory: India and Its Contradictions*. Princeton, NJ: Princeton University Press.

Durkheim, Émile. 2001. *The Elementary Forms of Religious Life*. Translated by Carol Cosman and Mark S. Cladis. Oxford: Oxford University Press.

Eberhardt, Nancy. 2006. *Imagining the Course of Life: Self-Transformation in a Shan Buddhist Community*. Honolulu: University of Hawai'i Press.

Engel, Davis, and Jaruwan Engel. 2010. *Tort, Custom, and Karma*. Chiang Mai: Silkworm Books.

Farmer, Paul. 1996. "On Suffering and Structural Violence: A View from Below." *Daedalus* 125 (1): 261–83.

———. 2003. *Pathologies of Power: Health, Human Rights, and the New War on the Poor*. Berkeley: University of California Press.

———. 2004. "An Anthropology of Structural Violence." *Current Anthropology* 45 (3): 305–25.

Farrely, Nicholas. 2012. "Exploitation and Escape: Journeys across the Burma-Thailand Frontier." In *Labour Migration and Human Trafficking in Southeast Asia: Critical Perspectives*, edited by Michelle Ford, Lenore Lyons, and William van Schendel, 130–48. New York: Routledge.

Fassin, Didier. 2009. "Another Politics of Life Is Possible." *Theory, Culture, Society* 26 (5): 44–60.

———. 2010. "Ethics of Survival: A Democratic Approach to the Politics of Life." *Humanity* 1 (1): 81–96.

———. 2012. *Humanitarian Reason: A Moral History of the Present.* Berkeley: University of California Press.

Ferguson, James. 2015. *Give a Man a Fish: Reflections on the New Politics of Distribution.* Durham, NC: Duke University Press.

Ferrarese, Estelle. 2016. "Vulnerability: A Concept with Which to Undo the World as It Is?" *Critical Horizons: A Journal of Philosophy and Social Theory* 17 (2): 149–59.

Foucault, Michel. 1973. *The Birth of the Clinic: An Archaeology of Medical Perception.* New York: Pantheon Books.

———. 1978. *The History of Sexuality.* Vol. 1. New York: Pantheon Books.

———. 2000. "Governmentality." In *The Essential Works of Foucault, 1954–1984,* vol. 3, *Power,* edited by James Faubion, 201–22. New York: New Press.

Franklin, Sarah. 1997. *Embodied Progress: A Cultural Account of Assisted Conception.* London: Routledge.

Fraser, Nancy. 2016. "Contradictions of Capital and Care." *New Left Review* 100:99–117.

Frohock, Fred M. 1986. *Special Care: Medical Decisions at the Beginning of Life.* Chicago: University of Chicago Press.

Gammeltoft, Tina. 2014. *Haunting Images: A Cultural Account of Selective Reproduction in Vietnam.* Berkeley: University of California Press.

Garcia, Angela. 2010. *The Pastoral Clinic: Addiction and Dispossession along the Rio Grande.* Berkeley: University of California Press.

Ghebreyesus, Tedros Adhanom. 2017. "All Roads Lead to Universal Health Coverage." *Lancet Global Health* 5 (9): e839-40.

Gilligan, Carol. 1982. *In a Different Voice: Psychological Theory and Women's Development.* Cambridge, MA: Harvard University Press.

Glenn, Evelyn Nakano. 2010. *Forced to Care: Coercion and Caregiving in America.* Cambridge, MA: Harvard University Press.

Golomb, Louis. 1984. "The Curer as Cultural Intermediary in Southern Thailand." *Social Science & Medicine* 18 (2): 111–15.

Gottret, Pablo, George Schieber, and Hugh Waters. 2008. *Good Practices in Health Financing: Lessons from Reforms in Low and Middle-Income Countries.* Washington, DC: World Bank.

Graeber, David. 2001. *Toward an Anthropological Theory of Value: The False Coin of Our Own Dreams.* New York: Palgrave.

Green, Linda. 2009. "The Fear of No Future: Guatemalan Migrants, Dispossession and Dislocation." *Anthropologica* 51 (2): 327–41.

Greenhalgh, Sarah, and Edwin A. Winckler. 2005. *Governing China's Population: From Leninist to Neoliberal Biopolitics*. Stanford: Stanford University Press.

Grosz, Elizabeth. 2005. *Time Travels: Feminism, Nature, Power*. Durham, NC: Duke University Press.

Gupta, Akhil. 1995. "Blurred Boundaries: The Discourse of Corruption, the Culture of Politics, and the Imagined State." *American Ethnologist* 22 (2): 375–402.

———. 2012. *Red Tape: Bureaucracy, Structural Violence, and Poverty in India*. Durham, NC: Duke University Press.

Haggard, Stephan, and Robert R. Kaufman. 2008. *Development, Democracy, and Welfare States: Latin America, East Asia, and Eastern Europe*. Princeton, NJ: Princeton University Press.

Hale, Ann. 1979. "A Reassessment of Northern Thai Matrilineages." *Mankind* 12 (2): 138–50.

Hall, Andy. 2011. "Migration and Thailand: Policy, Perspectives and Challenges." In *Thailand Migration Report*, edited by Jerrold W. Huguet and Aphichat Chamratrithirong, 17–35. Bangkok: IOM International Organization for Migration.

Handley, Paul. 2006. *The King Never Smiles: A Biography of Thailand's Bhumibol Adulyadej*. New Haven, CT: Yale University Press.

Hanks, Jane. 1963. *Maternity and Its Rituals in Bang Chan*. Ithaca, NY: Southeast Asia Program, Department of Asia Studies, Cornell University.

Hansen, Thomas and Finn Stepputat. 2006. "Sovereignty Revisited." *Annual Review of Anthropology* 35 (1): 295–315.

Haraway, Donna. (1985) 2003. "A Manifesto for Cyborgs: Science, Technology, and Socialist Feminism in the 1980s." In *The Haraway Reader*, edited by Donna J. Haraway, 7–46. New York: Routledge.

Harris, Joseph. 2012. "A Right to Health? Professional Networks, HIV/AIDS, and the Politics of Universal Health Care." PhD diss., University of Wisconsin–Madison.

———. 2013. "Uneven Inclusion: Consequences of Universal Healthcare in Thailand." *Citizenship Studies* 17 (1): 111–27.

———. 2015. "'Developmental Capture' of the State: Explaining Thailand's Universal Coverage Policy." *Journal of Health Politics, Policy and Law* 40 (1): 165–93.

———. 2017. *Achieving Access: Professional Movements and the Politics of Health Universalism*. Ithaca, NY: Cornell University Press.

Held, Virginia. 2006. *The Ethics of Care: Personal, Political, and Global*. Oxford: Oxford University Press.

Herzfeld, Michael. 2016. *Siege of the Spirits: Community and Polity in Bangkok*. Chicago: University of Chicago Press.

Hewison, Kevin. 2005. "Neo-Liberalism and Domestic Capital: The Political Outcomes of the Economic Crisis in Thailand." *Journal of Development Studies* 41 (2): 310–30.

———. 2017. "Reluctant Populists: Learning Populism in Thailand." *International Political Science Review* 38 (4): 426–40.

High, Holly. 2006. "Ritualising Residency: Territory Cults and a Sense of Place in Southern Lao PDR." *The Asia Pacific Journal of Anthropology* 7 (3): 251–63.

———. 2014. *Fields of Desire: Poverty and Policy in Laos*. Singapore: NUS Press.

Holmes, Seth. 2013. *Fresh Fruit, Broken Bodies: Migrant Farmworkers in the United States*. Berkeley: University of California Press.

Holt, John. 2009. *Spirits of the Place: Buddhism and Lao Religious Culture*. Honolulu: University of Hawai'i Press.

Honneth, Axel, Jacques Rancière, and Katia Genel. 2016. *Recognition or Disagreement: A Critical Encounter on the Politics of Freedom, Equality, and Identity*. New York: Columbia University Press.

Hull, Matthew. 2012a. "Documents and Bureaucracy." *Annual Review of Anthropology* 41 (1): 251–67.

———. 2012b. *Government of Paper: The Materiality of Bureaucracy in Urban Pakistan*. Berkeley: University of California Press.

Humphrey, Caroline. 2004. "Sovereignty." In *A Companion to the Anthropology of Politics*, edited by David Nugent and Joan Vincent, 418–36. Malden, MA: Blackwell.

———. 2012. "Hospitality and Tone: Holding Patterns for Strangeness in Rural Mongolia." *Journal of Royal Anthropological Institute*, n.s., 18:S63–75.

Ingold, Tim. 2011. *Being Alive: Essays on Movement, Knowledge and Description*. London: Routledge.

Irvine, Walter. 1982. "The Thai-Yuan 'Madman' and the 'Modernizing, Developing Thai Nation' as Bounded Entities under Threat: A Study in the Replication of a Single Image." PhD diss., University of London.

Jackson, Peter A. 1999a. "The Enchanting Spirit of Thai Capitalism: The Cult of Luang Phor Khoon and the Post-Modernization of Thai Buddhism." *South East Asia Research* 7 (1): 5–60.

———. 1999b. "Royal Spirits, Chinese Gods, and Magic Monks: Thailand's Boom-Time Religions of Prosperity." *South East Asia Research* 7 (3): 245–320.

———. 2004. "The Tapestry of Language and Theory: Reading Rosalind Morris on Post-Structuralism and Thai Modernity." *South East Asia Research* 12 (3): 337–77.

———. 2010. "Virtual Divinity: A 21st-Century Discourse of Thai Royal Influence." In *Saying the Unsayable: Monarchy and Democracy in Thailand*, edited by Søren Ivarsson and Lotte Isager, 29–60. Copenhagen: NIAS Press.

Jacob, Marie-Andree. 2007. "Form-Made Persons: Consent Forms as Consent's Blind Spot." *Political and Legal Anthropology Review* 30 (2): 249–68.

Johnson, Derina, Liberty Thawda, Sid Mone Thwe, and Hay Mar San. 2015. "Discovering Culturally Appropriate Psychosocial Care for Children and Young People." In *Trauma and Recovery on War's Border: A Guide for Global Health*

Workers, edited by Kathleen Allden and Nancy Murakami, 109–40. Hanover, NH: Dartmouth College Press.

Kamol Somvichian. 1976. "The Thai Political Culture and Political Development" In *Modern Thai Politics: From Village to Nation*, edited by Clark D. Neher, 153–69. Cambridge: Schenkman.

Karanikolos, Marian, Philipa Mladovsky, Jonathan Cylus, Sarah Thomson, Sanjay Basu, David Stuckler, Johan P. Mackenbach, and Martin McKee. 2013. "Financial Crisis, Austerity, and Health in Europe." *The Lancet* 381 (9874): 1323–31.

Katz, Pearl. 1981. "Ritual in the Operating Room." *Ethnology* 20 (4): 335–50.

Kaufman, Sharon. 2003. "Hidden Places, Uncommon Persons." *Social Science & Medicine* 56 (11): 2249–61.

Keane, Webb. 2016. *Ethical Life: Its Natural and Social Histories*. Princeton, NJ: Princeton University Press.

Kelly, Tobias. 2006. "Documented Lives: Fear and the Uncertainties of Law during the Second Palestinian Intifada." *Journal of the Royal Anthropological Institute* 12 (1): 89–107.

Kenner, Carole, and Judy Wright Lott. 2013. *Comprehensive Neonatal Nursing Care*. New York: Springer.

Keown, Damien. 1995. *Buddhism & Bioethics*. New York: St. Martin's.

Keshavjee, Salmaan. 2014. *Blind Spot: How Neoliberalism Infiltrated Global Health*. Berkeley: University of California Press.

Keyes, Charles. 1983. "Merit-Transference in the Karmic Theory of Popular Theravada Buddhism." In *Karma: An Anthropological Inquiry*, edited by Charles F. Keyes and E. Valentine Daniel, 261–86. Berkeley: University of California Press.

———. 2002. "Presidential Address: 'The Peoples of Asia': Science and Politics in the Classification of Ethnic Groups in Thailand, China, and Vietnam." *Journal of Asian Studies* 61 (4): 1163–203.

Keyes, Charles, and Valentine Daniel, eds. 1983. *Karma an Anthropological Inquiry*. Berkeley: University of California Press.

Kim, Jim Yong. 2013. "World Bank Group President Jim Yong Kim's Speech at World Health Assembly: Poverty, Health and the Human Future." World Bank, May 21. http://www.worldbank.org/en/news/speech/2013/05/21/world-bank-group-president-jim-yong-kim-speech-at-world-health-assembly.

Kittay, Eva Feder, and Ellen K. Feder. 2002. *The Subject of Care: Feminist Perspectives on Dependency*. Lanham, MD: Rowman & Littlefield.

Kleinman, Arthur. 2006. *What Really Matters: Living a Moral Life amidst Uncertainty and Danger*. Oxford: Oxford University Press.

———. 2015. "Care: In Search of a Health Agenda." *The Lancet* 386 (9990): 240–41.

———. 2017. "Presence." *The Lancet* 389 (10088): 2466–67.

Kuhonta, Erik. 2003. "The Political Economy of Equitable Development in Thailand." *American Asian Review* 21 (4): 69–108.

———. 2017. "The Politics of Health Care Reform in Thailand." In *Towards Universal Health Care in Emerging Economies*, edited by Ilcheong Yi, 91–118. Palgrave Macmillan, London.

Ladwig, Patrice. 2012. "Visitors from Hell: Transformative Hospitality to Ghosts in a Lao Buddhist Festival." *Journal of Royal Anthropological Institute*, n.s., 18:S90–102.

Laidlaw, James. 2000. "A Free Gift Makes No Friends." *Journal of the Royal Anthropological Institute* 6 (4): 617–34.

———. 2010. "Agency and Responsibility: Perhaps You Can Have Too Much of a Good Thing." In *Ordinary Ethics: Anthropology, Language, and Action*, edited by Michael Lambek, 143–64. New York: Fordham University Press.

Langford, Jean. 2005. "Spirits of Dissent: Southeast Asian Memories and Disciplines of Death." *Comparative Studies of South Asia, Africa and the Middle East* 25 (1): 161–76.

———. 2009. "Gifts Intercepted: Biopolitics and Spirit Debt." *Cultural Anthropology* 24 (4): 681–711.

Lantos, John D. 2001. *The Lazarus Case: Life-and-Death Issues in Neonatal Intensive Care*. Baltimore: Johns Hopkins University Press.

Leach, Edmund. 1982. *Social Anthropology*. Oxford: Oxford University Press.

Leiter, Karen, Voravit Suwanvanichkij, Ingrid Tamm, Vincent Iacopino, and Chris Beyrer. 2006. "Human Rights Abuses and Vulnerability to HIV/AIDS: The Experiences of Burmese Women in Thailand." *Health and Human Rights* 9 (2): 88–111.

Lévinas, Emmanuel. 1981. *Otherwise Than Being: Or, Beyond Essence*. Hague: Kluwer Boston.

Livingston, Julie. 2012. *Improvising Medicine: An African Oncology Ward in an Emerging Cancer Epidemic*. Durham, NC: Duke University Press.

Long, Debbi, Cynthia Hunter, and Sjaak van der Geest. 2008. "When the Field Is a Ward or a Clinic: Hospital Ethnography." *Anthropology & Medicine* 15 (2): 71–78.

Lyttleton, Chris. 1996. "Health and Development: Knowledge Systems and Local Practice in Rural Thailand." *Health Transition Review* 6 (1): 25–48.

Martin, Emily. 1987. *The Woman in the Body: A Cultural Analysis of Reproduction*. Boston: Beacon.

Mattingly, Cheryl. 2010. *The Paradox of Hope Journeys through a Clinical Borderland*. Berkeley: University of California Press.

Mauss, Marcel. (1954) 1990. *The Gift: The Form and Reason for Exchange in Archaic Societies*. Translated by W. D. Halls. London: Routledge.

———. (1960) 1992. "Techniques of the Body." In *Incorporations*, edited by Jonathan Crary and Sanford Kwinter, 455–77. New York: Zone.

McDaniel, Justin Thomas. 2011. *The Lovelorn Ghost and the Magical Monk: Practicing Buddhism in Modern Thailand*. New York: Columbia University Press.

McGuire, James. 2010. *Wealth, Health, and Democracy in East Asia and Latin America*. London: Cambridge.

McMorran, M. V. 1984. "Northern Thai Ancestral Cults: Authority and Aggression." *Mankind* 14 (4): 308–14.

Meehan, Katie, and Kendra Strauss, eds. 2015. *Precarious Worlds: Contested Geographies of Social Reproduction*. Athens: University of Georgia Press.

Mesman, Jessica. 2008. *Uncertainty and Medical Innovation in Neonatal Care: Experienced Pioneers in Neonatal Care*. Basingstoke, UK: Palgrave Macmillan.

Migrant Assistance Programme Foundation. 2012. *Regular Rights: Do Documents Improve Migrants' Lives?* Chiang Mai: MAP Foundation.

Mills, Mary Beth. 2012. "Thai Mobilities and Cultural Citizenship." *Critical Asian Studies* 44 (1): 85–112.

Mitchell, Katharyne, Cindi Katz, and Sallie A. Marston. 2004. *Life's Work: Geographies of Social Reproduction*. Hoboken, NJ: Wiley-Blackwell.

Mol, Annemarie. 2002. *The Body Multiple: Ontology in Medical Practice*. Durham, NC: Duke University Press.

———. 2008. *The Logic of Care: Health and the Problem of Patient Choice*. London: Routledge.

Mol, Annemarie, Ingunn Moser, and Jeannette Pols. 2010. *Care in Practice: On Tinkering in Clinics, Homes and Farms*. Bielefeld: Transcript.

Morris, Rosalind. 2000. *In the Place of Origins: Modernity and Its Mediums in Northern Thailand*. Durham, NC: Duke University Press.

Mougne, Christine. 1975. *An Ethnography of Reproduction: Changing Fertility Patterns in Northern Thailand*. London: School of Oriental and African Studies, University of London.

Muecke, Marjorie. 1979. "An Explication of 'Wind Illness' in Northern Thailand." *Culture, Medicine and Psychiatry* 3:267–300.

Muecke, Marjorie, and Wichit Srisuphan.1989. "Born Female: The Development of Nursing in Thailand." *Social Science & Medicine* 29 (5): 643–52.

Mulder, Niels. 1979. *Everyday Life in Thailand: An Interpretation*. Bangkok: Duang Kamol.

Nam, Illan. 2015. *Democratizing Health Care Welfare State Building in Korea and Thailand*. Houndmills: Palgrave Macmillan.

Nanchanok Wongsamuth. 2016. "Operating Within the Lawsuits." *Bangkok Post*, May 29.

Navaro-Yashin, Yael. 2007. "Make-Believe Papers, Legal Forms and the Counterfeit: Affective Interactions Between Documents and People in Britain and Cyprus." *Anthropological Theory* 7 (1): 79–98.

Nguyen, Vinh-Kim. 2010. *The Republic of Therapy: Triage and Sovereignty in West Africa's Time of AIDS*. Durham, NC: Duke University Press.

Nyein Nyein. 2013a. "Burmese Migrants to See Thai Work Eligibility Extended." *The Irrawaddy*, September 2.

———. 2013b. "Thai Police in Chiang Mai Arrest 200 Burmese Migrant Workers." *The Irrawaddy*, July 4.

Nyo Nyo. 2001. "Burmese Children in Thailand: Legal Aspects." *Legal Issues on Burma Journal* 10 (1): 51–56.

O'Toole, Bill. 2013a. "Migrants in Limbo as Thai Visas Expire." *Myanmar Times*, August 25.

———. 2013b. "Myanmar Workers Face Expiration of Work Visas." *Myanmar Times*, August 16.

Padmini Srikantiah, Massimo Ghidinelli, Damodar Bachani, Sanchai Chasombat, Esorom Daoni, Dyah Mustikawati, Do Nhan, Laxmi Pathak, Khin San, Mean Vun, Fujie Zhang, Ying-Ru Lo, and Jai Narain. 2010. "Scale-up of National Antiretroviral Therapy Programs: Progress and Challenges in the Asia Pacific Region." *AIDS* 24 (S3): S62–71.

Parry, James. 1989. "On the Moral Perils of Exchange." In *Money and the Morality of Exchange*, edited by J. Parry and M. Bloch, 64–93. Cambridge: Cambridge University Press.

Pasuk Phongpaichit, and Chris Baker. 2000. *Thailand's Crisis*. Chiang Mai: Silkworm Books.

———. 2009. *Thaksin*. Chiang Mai: Silkworm Books.

———. 2016. *Unequal Thailand: Aspects of Income, Wealth, and Power*. Singapore: NUS Press.

Petryna, Adriana. 2002. *Life Exposed*. Princeton, NJ: Princeton University Press.

Pinkaew Laungaramsri. 2014. "Contested Citizenship: Cards, Colors, and the Culture of Identification." In *Ethnicity, Borders, and the Grassroots Interface with the State: Studies on Southeast Asia*, edited by John A. Marston, 143–62. Chiang Mai: Silkworm Books.

Pitch Phongsawat. 2004. "Senthang prachathippatai lae kan prap tua khong rat thai nai rabop Thaksin [Democracy and state adjustment under Thaksin]." *Fa Dieo Kan* 2.

———. 2007. "Border Partial Citizenship, Border Towns, and Thai–Myanmar Cross-Border Development: Case Studies at the Thai Border Towns." PhD diss., University of California, Berkeley.

Pitrou, Perig. 2014. "Life as a Process of Making in the Mix Highlands (Oaxaca, Mexico): Towards a 'General Pragmatics' of Life." *Journal of the Royal Anthropological Institute* 21:86–105.

Poulsen, Anders. 1984. "Customs and Rites Connected with Pregnancy and Childbirth in a Northeastern Thai Village." *Asian Folklore Studies* 43:63–70.

———. 2007. *Childbirth and Tradition in Northeast Thailand: Forty Years of Development and Cultural Change*. Copenhagen: NIAS.

Povinelli, Elizabeth A. 2011. *Economies of Abandonment: Social Belonging and Endurance in Late Liberalism*. Durham, NC: Duke University Press.

Prachatai. 2017. "Problems of Thai Healthcare Bigger than Toon Can Solve." *Prachatai*, December 25.

Pranee Liamputtong. 2004. "Yu Duan Practices as Embodying Tradition, Modernity and Social Change in Chiang Mai, Northern Thailand." *Women & Health* 40 (1): 79–99.

Pranee Liamputtong, Niphattra Haritavorn, and Niyada Kiatying-Angsulee. 2013. "Women, Motherhood, and Living Positively: The Lived Experience of Thai Women Living with HIV/AIDS." In *Women, Motherhood and Living with HIV/AIDS: A Cross-Cultural Perspective*, edited by Pranee Liamputtong, 231–47. London: Springer.

Prapaporn Mongkhonvanit and Piya Hanvoravongchai. 2014. *The Impacts of Universalization: A Case Study on Thailand's Social Protection and Universal Health Coverage*. Geneva: UNRISD.

Puig de la Bellacasa, María. 2011. "Matters of Care in Technoscience: Assembling Neglected Things." *Social Studies of Science* 41 (1): 85–106.

———. 2017. *Matters of Care: Speculative Ethics in More Than Human Worlds*. Minneapolis: University of Minnesota Press.

Rabinow, Paul. 1992. "Artificiality and Enlightenment: From Sociology to Biosociality." In *Incorporations*, edited by Jonathan Crary and Sanford Kwinter, 234–52. New York: Zone Books.

Rancière, Jacques. 2004. "Who Is the Subject of the Rights of Man?" *South Atlantic Quarterly* 103 (2/3): 297–310.

———. 2011. "The Thinking of Dissensus: Politics and Aesthetics." In *Reading Rancière*, edited by Paul Bowman and Richard Stamp, 1–17. London: Continuum.

Rapeepong Suphanchaimat, Kanang Kantamaturapoj, Nareerut Pudpong, Weerasak Putthasri, and Anne Mills. 2016. "Health Insurance for People with Citizenship Problems in Thailand: A Case Study of Policy Implementation." *Health Policy and Planning* 31:229–38.

Rapeepong Suphanchaimat, Nareerut Pudpong, Phusit Prakongsai, Weerasak Putthasri, Johanna Hanefeld, and Anne Mills. 2019. "The Devil Is in the Detail: Understanding Divergence between Intention and Implementation of Health Policy for Undocumented Migrants in Thailand." *International Journal of Environmental Research and Public Health* 16 (6): 1–19.

Rapp, Rayna. 1999. *Testing Women, Testing the Fetus: The Social Impact of Amniocentesis in America*. New York: Routledge.

Reader, Soran. 2007. "The Other Side of Agency." *Philosophy* 82 (4): 579–604.

———. 2010. "Agency, Patiency, and Personhood." In *A Companion to the Philosophy of Action*, edited by Timothy O'Connor and Constantine Sandis, 200–208. Malden, MA: Wiley-Blackwell.

Redfield, Peter. 2005. "Doctors, Borders and Life in Crisis." *Cultural Anthropology* 20 (3): 328–61.

Reeves, Madeleine. 2013. "Clean Fake: Authenticating Documents and Persons in Migrant Moscow." *American Ethnologist* 40 (3): 508–24.

Reynolds, Craig J. 2005. "Power." In *Critical Terms for the Study of Buddhism*, edited by Donal S. Lopez Jr., 211–28. Chicago: University of Chicago Press.

Rice, Pranee Liamputtong, and Lenore Manderson, eds. 1996. *Maternity and Reproductive Health in Asian Societies*. Amsterdam: Harwood Academic.

Rigg, Jonathan. 2015. *Challenging Southeast Asian Development: The Shadows of Success*. London: Routledge.

Robinson, Fiona. 2011. *The Ethics of Care: A Feminist Approach to Human Security*. Philadelphia: Temple University Press.

Rose, Nikolas and Carlos Novas. 2004. "Biological Citizenship." In *Global Assemblages: Technology, Politics, and Ethics as Anthropological Problems*, edited by Aihwa Ong and Stephen J. Collier, 439–63. London: Blackwell.

Sakolsatayadorn Piyasakol. 2016. "Thailand: At the Forefront of Universal Health Coverage." Medium, December 12. https://medium.com/health-for-all/thailand-at-the-forefront-of-universal-health-coverage-d1bb9c0c3e79.

Samrit Srithamrongsawat, Ratanapron Wisessang, and Sarinthorn Ratjaroenkhajorn. 2010. *Financing Health Care for Migrants: A Case Study from Thailand*. Bangkok: International Organization for Migration.

Sansnee Jirojwong. 1996. "Health Beliefs and the Use of Antenatal Care among Pregnant Women in Southern Thailand." In *Maternity and Reproductive Health in Asian Societies*, edited by Pranee Liamputtong Rice and Lenore Manderson, 61–82. Amsterdam: Harwood Academic.

Scheper-Hughes, Nancy. 1992. *Death without Weeping: The Violence of Everyday Life in Brazil*. Berkeley: University of California Press.

———. 2008. "A Talent for Life: Reflections on Human Vulnerability and Resilience." *Ethnos* 73 (1): 25–56.

Scott, James. 1998. *Seeing Like a State: How Certain Schemes to Improve the Human Condition Have Failed*. New Haven, CT: Yale University Press.

Sen, Amartya. 2015. "Universal Healthcare: The Affordable Dream." *The Guardian*, January 6.

Seo, Bo Kyeong. 2019. "Populist Becoming: The Red Shirt Movement and Political Affliction in Thailand." *Cultural Anthropology* 34 (4): 555–79.

Sevenhuijsen, Selma. 1998. *Citizenship and the Ethics of Care: Feminist Considerations on Justice, Morality, and Politics*. London: Routledge.

Seymour, Jane. 2001. *Critical Moments: Death and Dying in Intensive Care*. Buckingham: Open University Press.

Singh, Bhrigupati. 2012. "The Headless Horseman of Central India: Sovereignty at Varying Thresholds of Life." *Cultural Anthropology* 27 (2): 383–407.

———. 2015. *Poverty and the Quest for Life: Spiritual and Material Striving in Rural India*. Chicago: University of Chicago Press.

Star, Susan Leigh. 1999. "The Ethnography of Infrastructure." *American Behavioral Scientist* 43 (3): 377–91.

Stasch, Rupert. 2009. *Society of Others: Kinship and Mourning in a West Papuan Place.* Berkeley: University of California Press.

Stevenson, Lisa. 2014. *Life Beside Itself: Imagining Care in the Canadian Arctic.* Berkeley: University of California Press.

Stonington, Scott. 2012. "On Ethical Locations: The Good Death in Thailand, Where Ethics Sit in Places." *Social Science & Medicine* 75 (5): 836–44.

Strathern, Marilyn. 1988. *The Gender of the Gift: Problems with Women and Problems with Society in Melanesia.* Berkeley: University of California Press.

———. 2004. *Partial Connections.* Walnut Creek, CA: AltaMira.

Street, Alice. 2012. "Seen by the State: Bureaucracy, Visibility and Governmentality in a Papua New Guinean Hospital." *Australian Journal of Anthropology* 23 (1): 1–21.

———. 2014. *Biomedicine in an Unstable Place: Infrastructure and Personhood in a Papua New Guinean Hospital.* Durham, NC: Duke University Press.

Street, Alice, and Simon Coleman. 2012. "Introduction: Real and Imagined Spaces." *Space and Culture* 15 (1): 4–17.

Supasit Pannarunothai, Direk Patmasiriwat, and Samrit Srithamrongsawat. 2004. "Universal Health Coverage in Thailand: Ideas for Reform and Policy Struggling." *Health Policy* 68 (1): 17–30.

Supon Limwattananon, Viroj Tangcharoensathien, Kanjana Tisayaticom, Tawekiat Boonyapaisarncharoen, and Phusit Prakongsai. 2012. "Why Has the Universal Coverage Scheme in Thailand Achieved a Pro-Poor Public Subsidy for Health Care?" *BMC Public Health* 12 (1): 1–11.

Supon Limwattananon, Viroj Tangcharoensathien, and Phusit Prakongsai. 2010. "Equity in Maternal and Child Health in Thailand." *Bulletin of the World Health Organization* 88 (6): 420–27.

Suriya Samutkhupt et al. 1996. *Song Jao Khao Phi: Watthakam Khorng Latthi-Phithi Lae Wikrittikankhorng Khwam-Than-Samai Nai Sangkhom Thai* [Spirit Medium Cult Discourses and Crises of Modernity in Thailand]. Nakhon Ratchasima, Thailand: Suranaree University of Technology.

Suwit Wibulpolprasert and Paichit Pengpaibon. 2003. "Integrated Strategies to Tackle the Inequitable Distribution of Doctors in Thailand: Four Decades of Experience." *Human Resources for Health* 1 (1): 1–12.

Symonds, Patricia. 1996. "Journey to the Land of Light: Birth among Hmong Women." In *Maternity and Reproductive Health in Asian Societies*, edited by Pranee Liamputtong Rice and Lenore Manderson, 103–24. Amsterdam: Harwood Academic.

Tambiah, Stanley Jeyaraja. 1970. *Buddhism and the Spirit Cults in North-East Thailand.* Cambridge: Cambridge University Press.

———. 1976. *World Conqueror and World Renouncer: A Study of Buddhism and Polity in Thailand against a Historical Background*. Cambridge: Cambridge University Press.

———. 1984. *The Buddhist Saints of the Forest and the Cult of Amulets: A Study in Charisma, Hagiography, Sectarianism, and Millennial Buddhism*. Cambridge: Cambridge University Press.

———. 1985. "A Thai Cult of Healing." In *Culture, Thought, and Social Action: An Anthropological Perspective*, edited by Stanley Jeyaraja Tambiah, 87–122. Cambridge, MA: Harvard University Press.

Tannenbaum, Nicola. 1995. *Who Can Compete against the World? Power-Protection and Buddhism in Shan Worldview*. Ann Arbor, MI: Association for Asian Studies.

Tapp, Nicholas. 2010. *The Impossibility of Self: An Essay on the Hmong Diaspora*. Berlin: LIT.

Taylor, Philip. 2004. *Goddess on the Rise: Pilgrimage and Popular Religion in Vietnam*. Honolulu: University of Hawai'i Press.

Termsak Chalermpalanupap. 2019. "Thailand's Recent Elections: Disappointments, Surprises and Non-Surprises." *Perspective* (31). https://www.iseas.edu.sg/images/pdf/ISEAS_Perspective_2019_31.pdf.

Tewarit Somkotra and Leizel P. Lagrada. 2008. "Payments for Health Care and Its Effect on Catastrophe and Impoverishment: Experience from the Transition to Universal Coverage in Thailand." *Social Science & Medicine* 67 (12): 2027–35.

Thak Chaloemtiarana. 1979. *Thailand: The Politics of Despotic Paternalism*. Ithaca, NY: Southeast Asia Program Publications.

Thelen, Tatjana. 2015. "Care as Social Organization: Creating, Maintaining and Dissolving Significant Relations." *Anthropological Theory* 15 (4): 497–515.

Thithimadee Arphattanano. 2012. "Education that Leads to Nowhere: Thailand's Education Policy for Children of Migrants." *International Journal of Multicultural Education* 14 (1): 1–15.

Ticktin, Miriam. 2011. *Casualties of Care: Immigration and the Politics of Humanitarianism in France*. Berkeley: University of California Press.

Torpey, John. 2000. *The Invention of the Passport: Surveillance, Citizenship, and the State*. Cambridge: Cambridge University Press.

Townsend, Kimberley, and Pranee Liamputtong Rice. 1996. "A Baby Is Born in Site 2 Camp: Pregnancy, Birth and Confinement among Cambodian Refugee Women." In *Maternity and Reproductive Health in Asian Societies*, edited by Pranee Liamputtong Rice and Lenore Manderson, 125–44. Amsterdam: Harwood Academic.

Toyota, Mika. 2005. "Subjects of the Nation without Citizenship: The Case of 'Hill Tribes' in Thailand." In *Multiculturalism in Asia*, edited by Will Kymlicka and Baogang He, 110–35. Oxford: Oxford University Press.

Tronto, Joan C. 1993. *Moral Boundaries: A Political Argument for an Ethic of Care*. New York: Routledge.

———. 2013. *Caring Democracy Markets, Equality, and Justice*. New York: New York University Press.

Tsing, Anna Lowenhaupt. 2015. *The Mushroom at the End of the World: On the Possibility of Life in Capitalist Ruins*. Princeton, NJ: Princeton University Press.

van der Geest, Sjaak. 2018. "Review of Care/Sorge: Construction, Reproduction, and Dissolution of Significant Relationships by Tatjana Thelen." *Medicine Anthropology Theory* 5 (4): 136–41.

van der Geest, Sjaak, and Kaja Finkler. 2004. "Hospital Ethnography: Introduction." *Social Science & Medicine* 59 (10): 1995–2001.

Van Esterik, Penny. 1996. "Nurturance and Reciprocity in Thai Studies." In *State Power and Culture in Thailand*, edited by E. Paul Durrenberger, 22–46. New Haven, CT: Yale Southeast Asia Studies.

———. 2000. *Materializing Thailand*. Oxford: Berg.

Vermeulen, Eric. 2004. "Dealing with Doubt: Making Decisions in a Neonatal Ward in the Netherlands." *Social Science & Medicine* 59 (10): 2071–85.

Viroj Tangcharoensathien, Anne Mills, and Toomas Palu. 2015. "Accelerating Health Equity: The Key Role of Universal Health Coverage in the Sustainable Development Goals." *BMC Medicine* 13:101.

Viroj Tangcharoensathien, Supon Limwattananon, Walaiporn Patcharanarumol, Jadej Thammatacharee. 2014. "Monitoring and Evaluating Progress towards Universal Health Coverage in Thailand." *PLoS Med* 11 (9): e1001726. https://doi.org/10.1371/journal.pmed.1001726.

Viroj Tangcharoensathien, Walaiporn Patcharanarumol, Por Ir, Syed Mohamed Aljunid, Ali Ghufron Mukti, Kongsap Akkhavong, Eduardo Banzon, Dang Boi Huong, Hasbullah Thabrany, and Anne Mills. 2011. "Health-Financing Reforms in Southeast Asia: Challenges in Achieving Universal Coverage." *The Lancet* 377 (9768): 863–73.

Viroj Tangcharoensathien, Woranan Witthayapipopsakul, Warisa Panichkriangkrai, Walaiporn Patcharanarumol, and Anne Mills. 2018. "Health Systems Development in Thailand: A Solid Platform for Successful Implementation of Universal Health Coverage." *The Lancet* 391 (10126): 1205–23.

Walaiporn Patcharanarumol, Viroj Tangcharoensathlen, Supon Limwattananon, Warsa Panlchkrlangkral, Kumaree Pachanee, Waraporn Poungkantha, Lucy Gilson, and Anne Mills. 2011. "Why and How Did Thailand Achieve Good Health at Low Cost." In *"Good Health at Low Cost" 25 Years On: What Makes a Successful Health System?*, edited by Dina Balabanova, Martin McKee, and Anne Mills, 193–233. London: London School of Hygiene and Tropical Medicine.

Walker, Andrew. 2012. *Thailand's Political Peasants: Power in the Modern Rural Economy*. Madison: University of Wisconsin Press.

Walther, Frans. 2005. "Withholding Treatment, Withdrawing Treatment, and Palliative Care in the Neonatal Intensive Care Unit." *Early Human Development* 81:965–72.
Weiner, Noga. 2009. "The Intensive Medical Care of Sick, Impaired, and Preterm Newborns in Israel and the Production of Vulnerable Neonatal Subjectivities." *Medical Anthropology Quarterly* 23 (3): 320–41.
Weisz, J. R., S. Suwanlert, W. Chaiyasit, and B. Walter. 1987. "Over- and Undercontrolled Referral Problems among Children and Adolescents from Thailand and the United States: The *Wat* and *Wai* of Cultural Differences." *Journal of Consulting and Clinical Psychology* 55 (5): 719–26.
Whittaker, Andrea. 1996. "Primary Health Services in Rural Thailand: Problems of Translating Policy into Practice." *Asian Studies Review* 20 (1): 68–83.
———. 2000. *Intimate Knowledge: Women and Their Health in North-East Thailand.* St. Leonards, N.S.W.: Allen & Unwin.
———. 2004. *Abortion, Sin and the State in Thailand.* New York: Routledge Curzon.
WHO/World Bank. 2015. *Tracking Universal Health Coverage: First Global Monitoring Report.* Geneva: World Health Organization.
———. 2017. *Tracking Universal Health Coverage: 2017 Global Monitoring Report.* Geneva: World Health Organization.
Widlok, Thomas. 2004. "Sharing by Default? Outline of an Anthropology of Virtue." *Anthropological Theory* 4 (1): 53–70.
Wijeyewardene, Gehan. 1981. "Scrubbing Scurf: Medium & Deity in Chiang Mai." *Mankind* 13 (1): 1–14.
———. 1986. *Place and Emotion in Northern Thai Ritual Behaviour*. Bangkok, Thailand: Pandora.
Wilkinson, Iain, and Arthur Kleinman. 2016. *A Passion for Society: How We Think about Human Suffering*. Berkeley: University of California Press.
Willen, Sarah. 2005. "Birthing 'Invisible' Children: State Power, NGO Activism, and Reproductive Health among 'Illegal Migrant' Workers in Tel Aviv, Israel." *Journal of Middle East Women's Studies* 1 (2): 55–88.
———. 2012. "How Is Health-Related 'Deservingness' Reckoned? Perspectives from Unauthorized Im/migrants in Tel Aviv." *Social Science and Medicine* 74 (6): 812–21.
Wilson, Ara. 2008. "The Sacred Geography of Bangkok's Markets." *International Journal of Urban and Regional Research* 32 (3): 631–42.
———. 2010. "Medical Tourism in Thailand." In *Asian Biotech: Ethics and Communities of Fate*, edited by Aihwa Ong and Nancy N. Chen, 118–43. Durham, NC: Duke University Press.
———. 2011. "Foreign Bodies and National Scales: Medical Tourism in Thailand." *Body & Society* 17 (2–3): 121–37.

Wind, Gitte. 2008. "Negotiated Interactive Observation: Doing Fieldwork in Hospital Settings." *Anthropology & Medicine* 15 (2): 79–89.

Worawan Chandoevwit. 2005. "Financing Universal Health-Care Coverage." *TDRI Quarterly Review* 20 (3): 14–19.

World Health Organization's Global Health Workforce Statistics. n.d. "Nurses and Midwives (per 1,000 people)." World Health Organization's Global Health Workforce Statistics. Accessed March 19, 2019. https://data.worldbank.org/indicator/SH.MED.NUMW.P3?locations=TH.

Yang, Bryant Yuan Fu. 2007. "Life and Death Away from the Golden Land: The Plight of Burmese Migrant Workers in Thailand." *Asian-Pacific Law and Policy Journal* 8 (2): 485–535.

Thai-Language Source

พระยา สุนทรพิพิธ Phraya Sunthonphiphit. (1973) 2516. "วิญญาณ (Spirit) แห่งนักปกครอง (กรุงเทพฯ: อนุสรณ์ในงานพระราชทานเพลิงศพพระยาสุนทรพิพิธ)." In *Winyan [Spirit] haeng nak pokkhrong* [Spirit of the Governor]. Bangkok: Cremation Volume for Phraya Sunthonphiphit.

INDEX

Page numbers in italics refer to illustrations.

abortion, 111, 125, 156n5. *See also* antenatal care; births; infants; neonatal intensive care units (NICU); reproduction (medical)
Agamben, Giorgio, 59
aid (state), 19, 57, 144
AIDS, 128, 130, 135, 137, 153n8
America, 32
antenatal care: access to, 63, 137, 142, 155n13; and compliance, 58, 60, 64–67, 98; and documentation, 60, 64, 72
antiretroviral treatment, 129–30, 137, 150n2, 153n8
ap duean, 103–4
asceticism, 102, 120, 130–31, 134, 158n6, 158n9, 160n13. *See also* mothers; rituals; spirits (deities)
asphyxia, 82, 111
Auyero, Javier, 48

babies. *See* infants
bat samsip bat (30-baht Card), 41–47, 53, 64, 150n6, 152n1
Bhumibol Adulyadej (king), 44, 144, 153n6
biomedicine, 5, 14, 18, 24–29, 32, 80–81, 86, 93–98, 130, 135
biopolitics, 8, 15, 17, 60, 82, 92, 147
biopower, 8–9, 15
births: complications of, 69, 78, 82, 98, 101–2, 104, 111, 114; and documentation, 59–60, 67, 69–70, 72–74, 75, 81, 83, 136; and migrants, 75, 155n10. *See also* antenatal care; documentation (political); infants; mothers; neonatal intensive care units (NICU); rituals
blessings. *See* rituals; spirit mediums
bodies, 3–4, 6, 16, 20. *See also* care (medical); elicitation (care); feet; heads (body); nurses
Bourdieu, Pierre, 51–52, 56, 98
Buddhism, 17, 87, 100–102, 118, 122, 127, 131–38, 152n19, 153n5, 153n11, 156n7, 159n4, 159n6, 160n13. *See also* spirit mediums; Theravada

bureaucracy, 7, 18, 38, 60, 70, 74, 77, 91, 155n14. *See also* documentation (political); governing; politics
Burma (Myanmar), 15, 19, 19–20, 52, 56, 58, 101–5, 110, 130, 136–37. *See also* the Shan (migrants)

cancer, 24–30, 42, 49–50, 130
care: and belonging, 13, 16, 87, 142, 145, 147; challenges of, 6, 57, 79, 85; circuitry of, 18, 82–86, 90, 120, 140; and compassion, 86, 157n13; and compliance, 14, 24, 49, 70; dailiness of, 4–5, 13, 29, 130; definitions of, 5, 7–8, 37; demands of, 91, 109, 142; and dependency, 36, 87, 93; ethics of, 6, 9, 31, 37–38, 57, 79, 93, 138, 144, 152n19; experience of, 7, 9, 95, 109, 121, 141; and gender, 37, 150n5, 157n13; as generative, 6, 8, 20–21; importance of, 6, 145; and karma, 56, 147; methods of, 28, 51, 90–91, 119, 146; multiplicity of, 98–99, 135; necessity of, 13, 48, 148; and obligation, 13, 28–30, 32, 54, 69, 82, 85, 99, 144–45, 148; and patients, 14, 18–19, 142; potentialities of, 6, 20, 22, 141, 147; practices of, 9, 14, 27, 38, 79, 115; provision of, 12, 18, 30, 32, 37, 142, 145, 147; relationships of, 15, 49, 92, 139, 143; and spirituality, 16, 159n4; visions of, 21, 79–80, 108, 141–42; and vulnerability, 92, 139, 142. *See also* elicitation (care); families; hospitals (district); insurance (health); mothers; nurses; spirits (deities); Universal Health Coverage (UHC)
caregivers. *See* families; hospitals (district)
Cavarero, Adriana, 157n13
ceremonies. *See* births; rituals; spirit mediums
chang yai, 158n12
chants. See *khatha*
chaoban, 34
charity, 44–46, 48–49, 54, 56. *See also* aid (state); hospitals (district); nurses
chemotherapy, 24, 27–28, 49. *See also* cancer
childbirth. *See* births
children, 35, 75, 156n18. *See also* education; families; fathers; infants; mothers
chronic obstructive pulmonary disease (COPD), 35
chumchon, 34
citizenship (Thai): dreams of, 73, 136; effects of, 30, 73, 77; and eligibility, 54, 58, 73–74, 155n9; and exclusion, 54, 57–58. *See also* births; documentation (political); governing; infants; migrants
Civil Registration Act (2008), 74
Civil Servant Medical Benefit Scheme, 30, 82
Cohen, Lawrence, 74
community outreach, 35–37. *See also* hospitals (district); marginalized groups; nurses
Compulsory Migrant Health Insurance (CMHI), 28, 81, 121, 150n6, 155n12. *See also* insurance (health)

Das, Veena, 110, 119
Day, Sophie, 161n16
death: and ceremonies, 91–92, 140; decisions about, 38, 79–93, 141, 143, 154n14; and spirituality, 16, 84, 88–91, 128, 139. *See also* infants; karma; neonatal intensive care units (NICU)

debt. *See* economics; hospitals (district); *kreng jai*
deportations, 61–62. *See also* documentation (political); migrants; policing; work permits
depression, 71, 107–8
development (economic), 11–12, 24. *See also* economics; hospitals (district); politics
"development king," 44
diagnoses, 28, 49, 71, 89, 105–9, 121, 147, 151n12. See also *lom phit duean*
dialysis, 35, 39, 57, 121. *See also* kidneys
diet, 5, 96–102, 131, 158n6. See also *lom phit duean*
diseases. See *specific diseases*
doctors. *See* health care; hospitals (district); nurses
documentation (political): and birth, 14, 59–60, 67, 69–71, 75–76, 85; challenges of, 60, 73; and citizenship, 59, 85, 151n9, 155n12; and hospitals, 28–30, 89; importance of, 63, 73, 75, 136, 155n15; and migrants, 19, 28, 58, 73, 154n8; and permits, 52, 58, 64, 74, 77, 116; processes of, 14, 61–62, 74, 121, 155n14; and safety, 73–74, 77. *See also* citizenship (Thai); insurance (health); migrants
"Do Not Resuscitate," 79, 82, 84, 86, 88–90, 111. *See also* death; infants; neonatal intensive care units (NICU)

economics: and crisis, 11–12, 23, 82; experience of, 20, 130, 151n13; and health care, 7, 18, 35; limits of, 12, 29, 56, 117. *See also* governing; hospitals (district)
education, 44, 68, 155n15
elicitation (care): as agreement, 57, 146, 158n8; and belonging, 60, 79, 117, 142; definitions of, 6, 13; and infants, 79–80, 82, 92; methods of, 6, 19, 60; power of, 82, 142, 146; presence as, 14, 19, 36, 62–63, 142, 147–48; relationships of, 16–17, 36, 139, 141, 143; and vulnerability, 92, 95; waiting as, 13–14, 25–26, 39–41, 47–48, 51, 55, 135, 146, 161n16. *See also* care; marginalized groups; spirits (deities)
England, 49–50
epilepsy, 105

families: abandonment by, 29, 84–85, 87–88, 90, 105–6, 109, 140; as carers, 3–5, 28, 101, 115, 124, 141; concerns of, 27–28, 49, 114, 124; crises of, 6, 59, 104–5, 113, 129; and nurses, 4, 35. *See also* fathers; hospitals (district); infants; mothers; nurses
family planning, 63. *See also* antenatal care; reproduction (medical)
fathers: and births, 26, 69, 79, 83–84; care by, 56, 135; roles of, 28, 51, 100–101, 129
feet, 3–6, 78, 120, 141. *See also* bodies
Ferguson, James, 146
Foucault, Michel, 8, 26

Garcia, Angela, 138
gender, 8, 20, 37, 60, 102, 141, 147. *See also* fathers; mothers
ghosts. *See* spirits (deities)
governing, 34, 36–38, 69, 74, 77, 81, 143–44, 155n15, 161n1. *See also* bureaucracy; economics; politics
gratitude, 18, 41–47, 50, 56. See also *kreng jai*
grief. *See* death; families
Gupta, Akhil, 9

Handley, Paul, 44
Hanks, Jane, 100
hap khan, 130
Harris, Joseph, 42
heads (body), 5–6, 28, 84, 104, 108, 113
healing. *See* care
health care: access to, 22, 55, 61, 65, 143, 145, 155n12; distribution of, 21, 56, 147, 155n12; portrayals of, 19, 22, 39, 45, 55, 161n5; and privatization, 32, 145, 153n3; provisions of, 18, 47, 51, 153n6; as right, 10, 14, 29, 32, 44, 50, 143, 161n1. *See also* care; elicitation (care); hospitals (district); insurance (health); Universal Health Coverage (UHC)
health insurance. *See* insurance (health)
Health Insurance for People with Citizenship Problems (HIS-PCP), 151n10, 151n13, 155n12
Health Security Act, 53
Highlanders Card, 73, 156n16
HIV, 128, 130, 135, 137, 153n8
Holt, John, 127
home visits, 34–36, 70, 108. *See also* community outreach; nurses
Homo Sacer (Agamben), 59
hospitals (district): bills from, 28–29, 52–53, 89, 104, 121; as borderlands, 23–24, 151n13; budgets of, 30, 32–33, 50, 53, 113, 143–44, 151n12, 153n8; capacities of, 24–26, 29–30, 79–80, 142, 153n3; and collaboration, 24, 118, 144; and community outreach, 34–35, 37–38, 144; dangers of, 77, 110–12, 115; and discrimination, 77, 114; ethics of, 18, 22, 27, 53, 87; expansion of, 6, 19, 144, 152n1; and governing, 18, 25–30, 33–34, 67; limitations of, 10, 48, 108, 120–22; reliance upon, 40–41, 54; sovereignty of, 26, 28, 32–33, 38, 48, 69; and specialized care, 39, 49, 66, 98; and spirituality, 118, 130; transportation between, 27–28, 80–81, 121; travel to, 4, 67, 70, 81, 101, 112–13, 115, 140; and waiting, 51, 66, 94. *See also* care; health care; Intensive Care Unit (ICU); neonatal intensive care units (NICU); nurses
hospitals (private), 7, 24, 39, 49–51, 53, 65, 152n1, 153n3, 161n3. *See also* hospitals (district); income
humor (bodies), 97, 109, 157n4, 158n6. See also *lom phit duean*
Humphrey, Caroline, 38
hypoxia, 75, 78. *See also* births; infants; neonatal intensive care units (NICU)

income, 3, 6, 10–11, 20, 39, 129. *See also* economics; families; fathers; laborers; marginalized groups; migrants
indebtedness, 45–46, 48, 52–54, 56–57. *See also* hospitals (district); income; *kreng jai*; marginalized groups; migrants
inequalities, 7–15, 55, 82, 102, 141, 145–46. See also *kreng jai*; marginalized groups; migrants
infants: agency of, 82–86; care for, 20, 35, 53, 59, 75, 81–85, 90, 92; and citizenship, 58–59, 74, 85; and insurance, 89; and karma, 86, 89, 154n1; and personhood, 79, 82, 91–92; prematurity of, 20, 52, 156n6; vulnerability of, 14, 19–20, 33, 79, 83, 85, 92–93, 99, 138, 142. *See also* antenatal care; citizenship (Thai); death; karma; mothers; neonatal intensive care units (NICU); nurses

insurance (health), 4, 10, 38, 53, 55–56, 64, 143
Intensive Care Unit (ICU), 3. *See also* neonatal intensive care units (NICU)
Isan, 129

karma, 57, 84, 86, 91, 98–99, 102, 104, 156n7. *See also* Buddhism; death; infants; *lom phit duean*
Keown, Damien, 87
khan, 130
khatha, 132, *133*, 134
khwan, 16
kidneys, 115, 120–22, 124. *See also* dialysis
Kim, Jim Yong, 10
kreng jai, 49–52, 54–57, 67, 140, 147. *See also* hospitals (district); indebtedness; nurses
kuman thohng, 138

laborers: bodies of, 3; bodily risk of, 3–5; exploitation of, 61, 94–95; health insurance of, 4; income of, 39; rights of, 62; rituals of, 96; vulnerability of, 94, 115; wages of, 113
lak phoy, 97
liang, 152n18
lom phit duean, 96–97, 99, 103–5, 107, 109, 156n7, 157n4–157n5
loyalty, 28, 43, 56. *See also* families; hospitals (district); marginalized groups; monarchy (Thai); politics; Thailand

Mahidol Adulyadej (prince), 44
marginalized groups: and care, 9, 20, 75, 141; desires of, 13, 47–48; and insurance, 24, 28–31, 55; legitimacy of, 14, 31, 75; and politics, 7, 19, 30, 41; and poverty, 19, 43; survival of, 9, 12, 49; vulnerability of, 8, 11, 18, 39–40, 157n2. *See also* migrants; Myanmar; the poor (socioeconomic group); the Shan (migrants)
Mauss, Marcel, 48
medication, 28, 35, 39, 78, 82–86, 103–9, 114, 130
mental illness, 24, 108–9. See also *lom phit duean*
migrants: and birth, 63, 69, 82, 155n10; burdens of, 68, 120, 122; and care, 14, 69, 79, 142, 145; and displacement, 60, 109, 124, 154n8; and documentation, 19, 58, 60, 62–63, 70, 75, 82, 154n8, 155n14; and families, 3, 59, 63, 77, 95, 110, 140; as laborers, 4, 23, 102, 116, 155n12, 158n12; and legality, 61, 69, 85, 116; and poverty, 61, 121; rights of, 54, 77, 117; status of, 59, 72–73; vulnerability of, 94, 109–10, 112–13, 116–17, 137–38, 146, 156n17. *See also* citizenship (Thai); documentation (political); marginalized groups; the Shan (migrants)
militarism, 11, 19, 102, 143–44, 154n8. *See also* monarchy (Thai); policing; politics
Ministry of Interior, 154n8
Ministry of Public Health, 33, 144
monarchy (Thai), 10–11, 19, 41, 44–46, 144, 153n6. *See also* governance; politics; Thailand
Mongkut (king), 44
Moore, Michael, 32
mothers: absence of, 78, 82–83, 87–88, 90; and antenatal care, 19, 155n15; compassion of, 52, 100, 157n13; fears of, 99–100, 102, 106, 128, 136; rituals of, 58, 96–97, 137; vulnerability of, 94–96, 99, 112. *See also* families
Mus, Paul, 127

Myanmar, 15, 19, 19–20, 52–65, 74, 101–5, 110, 130, 136–37. *See also* the Shan (migrants)
Myanmar Citizenship Act, 156n17

National Economic and Social Development Plans (Thai), 11
National Health Security Office (NHSO), 29–30, 32–33
neonatal intensive care units (NICU), 33, 52–53, 75–93, 111, 119, 142, 148. *See also* births; death; families; fathers; infants; karma; mothers; nurses
1997 crisis (Thailand), 11–12, 47, 153. *See also* economics; politics; Thailand
nurses: capacities of, 33, 39, 67, 82, 86–87, 89, 93, 140, 151n7; care by, 64, 66–67, 92; choices of, 90, 93; and emotions, 70, 90–91, 103, 111; ethics of, 29, 33, 135; as family, 4, 29, 35, 83, 88–89, 112–14; and medical professionals, 18, 39, 51, 56, 114–15, 119, 142, 144, 151n10; and outreach, 34–36; relationships with, 19, 35, 60, 67–68, 70, 79, 114, 130, 155n13; role of, 34, 37, 69, 90–91, 142, 152n15; sense of duty of, 29, 36, 68–69, 78, 83, 85–86, 88, 91–92, 112, 148. *See also* care; families; hospitals (district); insurance (health)

passports, 62
patiency, 13, 85
personhood. *See* documentation (political); elicitation (care); infants; marginalized groups; migrants
Phalang Pracharat, 161n4
Phra Thep, 45
physiotherapy, 114, 130
ploi, 89, 157n8
policing, 9, 61, 73, 107–8, 136–37, 144, 154n8. *See also* documentation (political); marginalized groups; migrants; militarism
politics: and benevolence, 44, 48; and conflict, 40, 48, 63, 143–44; evolution of, 10, 43, 146–47, 152n19; and health care, 18, 30–31, 42, 60, 146; and legitimacy, 8–10, 19, 22, 38; and obligation, 31, 37, 54; and power, 11, 41, 55; and radicalism, 11, 13, 43, 158n14
the poor (socioeconomic group), 43, 55, 57. *See also* income; marginalized groups; migrants; urban-rural divide
postpartum restrictions. *See* births; *lak phoy*; *lom phit duean*; mothers; rituals; spirits (deities); *yu duean*
poverty, 120, 129, 141, 143, 148. *See also* income; marginalized groups; migrants
Povinelli, Elizabeth, 13
power, 9–10, 15, 17, 26, 50–51, 55–56
Prayuth Chan-Ocha, 161n4
pregnancy. *See* antenatal care; births; depression; mothers; neonatal intensive care units (NICU); reproduction (medical); the Shan (migrants)
privatization. *See* economics; health care
psychiatry, 105, 107–9
public health, 8, 11, 39–40, 54, 124, 141. *See also* health care
Puig de la Bellacasa, Maria, 149n3
pulmonary hypertension, 89

rape, 106, 108, 137. *See also* violence
rap khan, 130, 160n10
Reader, Soran, 13
reciprocity, 16, 40, 49, 57, 147. *See also* care; elicitation; karma; *kreng jai*

refugees, 9, 19, 59, 61, 82, 145. *See also* Burma (Myanmar); migrants; militarism; policing; the Shan (migrants)
renal replacement therapy, 39, 57, 121, 150n2, 150n6. *See also* kidneys
reproduction, 19, 60, 63, 70, 80
respiratory distress, 82, 84, 88. *See also* infants; neonatal intensive care units (NICU)
Reynolds, Craig, 17
rituals, 5, 16, 59, 96–100, 118–19, 125–30, 139, 154n1, 159n5. *See also* families; infants; karma; *lom phit duean*; mothers; spirits (deities)
royal family. *See* monarchy (Thai)
Rural Doctors Society, 149n11
rural-urban divide, 11, 22, 24–25, 48, 82, 94, 119

schizophrenia, 105
Sen, Amartya, 10
the Shan (migrants): and antenatal care, 68, *71*, 75–78, 81; and care, 63–65, 67–68, 110, *126*, 128; and children, 63, 66–67, 74, 156n17; desires of, 59–60, 63, 65, 100; and families, 20, 60, 68, 70, 94, 147–48; hardships of, 61, 72, 95, 100–101, 103, 125, 143; spirituality of, 127, 154n1; vulnerability of, 68, 105, 116, 120, 136. *See also* Buddhism; citizenship (Thai); documentation (political); marginalized groups; migrants; militarism; Myanmar; policing
Shan State, 15, 19–20, 52, 56, 58, 130, 136, *xvii*
shrine, *131*. *See also* Buddhism; spirit mediums
Sicko (Moore), 32
Singh, Bhrilgupati, 127
Sirindhorn, Maha Chakri (princess), 45
soldiers, 44, 101–2. *See also* Burma (Myanmar); policing
sovereignty, 15, 32–33, 38, 46, 51, 59, 82. *See also* economics; hospitals (district); politics; spirits (deities)
spirit mediums, 124, 127–32, 135, 154n1, 159n4, 160n11
spirits (deities): and danger, 119, 127, 139; desires of, 130–31, 135–36, 159n6; existence of, 119–20, 127–28, 132, 159n4, 159n7, 160n7; and healing, 16, 124, 135, 139; power of, 16–17, 20, 97, 118, 126–28, 139; protection by, 20, 122, 124–26, 129–30, 132, 134, 138; relationships with, 125, 134, 143; and rituals, 16, 98, 126, 132; and worship, 16, 132, 134–35. *See also* rituals
Stevenson, Lisa, 9
Street, Alice, 14, 155n14
suicide, 106, 125
surgery, 4, 24, 27, 42, 49–50, 54, 111, 121–22, 130. *See also* hospitals (district); insurance (health)

Tambiah, Stanley, 127
Tannenbaum, Nicola, 17
taxes, 45, 50, 144, 152n3. *See also* bureaucracy
technology, 8, 14, 16, 29, 79. *See also* biomedicine
"Ten-Year Card," 58
Thailand: culture of, 6, 15, 17, 21, 75; economics of, 11, 23–24, 55; geography of, 18–19, 23, *xvi*, *xvii*; health care in, 6–7, 9–11, 24–25, 143, 149n9; history of, 16–17, 38; monarchy of, 10, 41, 44, 46; politics of, 10, 40, 43, 143–44, 152n19; social contexts of, 8–10, 23, 50–51, 74, 109, 134, 158n6,

Thailand (*continued*)
158n13; spirituality in, 16, 119, 126–27, 134, 159n4. *See also* citizenship (Thai); economics; monarchy (Thai)
Thai Rak Thai Party (politics), 11, 41
Thak Chaloemtiarana, 44
Thaksin Shinawatra, 11–12, 19, 41–43, 45–46, 144
Theravada, 17, 44, 100, 153n5, 153n11
30-baht Card, 41–47, 53, 64, 150n6, 152n1
Tronto, Joan, 8
tuberculosis, 110–11, 116

United Nations, 145
United States, 32
Universal Health Coverage (UHC): access to, 19, 25, 29–30, 43, 92, 142, 150n2; debates of, 30, 46, 143–44; expansion of, 12, 21, 24, 41–42, 55, 120, 141, 143, 153n3, 161n3; experience of, 40–41, 57; limitations of, 39, 49, 153n8; promises of, 6, 31, 47, 55, 145, 151n9, 151n10, 151n12
urban-rural divide, 11, 22, 24–25, 48, 82, 94, 119

violence, 19–20, 56, 95, 102–10, 117, 127, 138, 143, 157n2

welfare (political), 8, 12, 44–49, 55, 61, 66, 127, 145–47. *See also* bureaucracy; governing; Universal Health Coverage (UHC)
Whittaker, Andrea, 98
wind afflictions, 96–97, 99, 102–5, 107, 109, 156n7, 157n4–157n5. See also *lom phit duean*
work permits, 61, 63. *See also* documentation (political); laborers; migrants
World Bank, 10
World Health Assembly, 10

Yingluck Shinawatra, 144
yu duean, 96, 98, 100. See also *lom phit duean*; postpartum restrictions

New Perspectives in Southeast Asian Studies

The Burma Delta: Economic Development and Social Change on an Asian Rice Frontier, 1852–1941
MICHAEL ADAS

Rise of the Brao: Ethnic Minorities in Northeastern Cambodia during Vietnamese Occupation
IAN G. BAIRD

Of Beggars and Buddhas: The Politics of Humor in the "Vessantara Jataka" in Thailand
KATHERINE A. BOWIE

Voices from the Plain of Jars: Life under an Air War, second edition
Edited by FRED BRANFMAN with essays and drawings by LAOTIAN VILLAGERS

A Reckoning: Philippine Trials of Japanese War Criminals
SHARON W. CHAMBERLAIN

From Rebellion to Riots: Collective Violence on Indonesian Borneo
JAMIE S. DAVIDSON

Feeding Manila in Peace and War, 1850–1945
DANIEL F. DOEPPERS

The Floracrats: State-Sponsored Science and the Failure of the Enlightenment in Indonesia
ANDREW GOSS

In Plain Sight: Impunity and Human Rights in Thailand
TYRELL HABERKORN

Revolution Interrupted: Farmers, Students, Law, and Violence in Northern Thailand
TYRELL HABERKORN

Philippine Sanctuary: A Holocaust Odyssey
BONNIE M. HARRIS

Amazons of the Huk Rebellion: Gender, Sex, and Revolution in the Philippines
VINA A. LANZONA

Dreams of the Hmong Kingdom: The Quest for Legitimation in French Indochina, 1850–1960
MAI NA M. LEE

The Government of Mistrust: Illegibility and Bureaucratic Power in Socialist Vietnam
KEN MACLEAN

An Anarchy of Families: State and Family in the Philippines
EDITED BY ALFRED W. MCCOY

Policing America's Empire: The United States, the Philippines, and the Rise of the Surveillance State
ALFRED W. MCCOY

Vietnam's Strategic Thinking during the Third Indochina War
KOSAL PATH

The Hispanization of the Philippines: Spanish Aims and Filipino Responses, 1565–1700
JOHN LEDDY PHELAN

Pretext for Mass Murder: The September 30th Movement and Suharto's Coup d'État in Indonesia
JOHN ROOSA

Hamka's Great Story: A Master Writer's Vision of Islam for Modern Indonesia
JAMES R. RUSH

Eliciting Care: Health and Power in Northern Thailand
BO KYEONG SEO

Dead in the Water: Global Lessons from the World Bank's Hydropower Project in Laos
Edited by BRUCE SHOEMAKER and WILLIAM ROBICHAUD

The Social World of Batavia: Europeans and Eurasians in Colonial Indonesia, second edition
JEAN GELMAN TAYLOR

Everyday Economic Survival in Myanmar
ARDETH MAUNG THAWNGHMUNG